Foucault, Health and Medicine

The reception of Michel Foucault's work in the social sciences and humanities has been phenomenal. Foucault's concepts and methodology have encouraged new approaches to old problems and have opened up new lines of enquiry. The study of health and medicine is no exception and his influence is so profound here that few topics in the field are discussed without some reliance on his work. *Foucault, Health and Medicine* assesses the contribution of Foucault's work in this area.

The foreword offers some reflections on Foucault's contribution to medical sociology as a whole. Part I problematises Foucault's work, examining the different 'readings' to which it lends itself. Part II deals with his concept of 'discourse' and explores some of its applications: the study of personality disorder and the problem of the 'dangerous individual', the study of the problem of child mental health, and the critique of the 'medicalisation' thesis. Part III turns to the analysis of the body and the self, major themes in Foucault's work. The implications of Foucault's concepts for feminist research on embodiment and gendered subjectivities are explored, and the notion of 'biopower' is considered in the context of health education. Finally, Part IV explores the application of Foucault's concept of governmentality to the analysis of health policy, health promotion and the consumption of health. Common themes in these chapters include the emergence of risk culture, the concept of the enterprising self and the role of expertise in liberal technologies of government.

Alan Petersen is Senior Lecturer in Sociology at Murdoch University, Western Australia. **Robin Bunton** is Senior Lecturer in Social Policy at the University of Teesside, Middlesbrough.

Foucault, Health and Medicine

Edited by Alan Petersen and Robin Bunton

Foreword by Bryan S. Turner

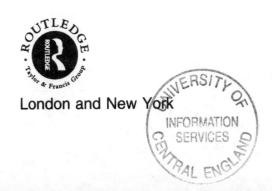

London and New York

First published 1997
by Routledge
11 New Fetter Lane, London EC4P 4EE

Simultaneously published in the USA and Canada
by Routledge
29 West 35th Street, New York, NY 10001

Reprinted 1998, 2000

Routledge is an imprint of the Taylor & Francis Group

© 1997 Alan Petersen and Robin Bunton, selection and
editorial matter; individual chapters, the contributors

Typeset in Times by
LaserScript, Mitcham, Surrey
Printed and bound in Great Britain by
Clays Ltd, St Ives plc

British Library Cataloguing in Publication Data
A catalogue record for this book is available from the British
Library

Library of Congress Cataloging in Publication Data
A catalog record for this book is available from the Library
of Congress

ISBN 0–415–15177–5 (hbk)
ISBN 0–415–15178–3 (pbk)

Contents

Contributors

David Armstrong is Reader in Sociology as Applied to Medicine, Department of General Practice, at the United Medical and Dental Schools of Guy's and St Thomas's Hospitals (UMDS).

Robin Bunton is Principal Lecturer in Social Policy in the School of Human Studies at the University of Teesside and works as a member of the Centre for the Study of Adult Life (C-SAL) at the University.

Liz Eckermann is Senior Lecturer in Sociology of Health and Illness, and Director of the Centre for the Body and Society, at Deakin University, Geelong, Victoria, Australia. Recent publications include 'Self-starvation and binge-purging: embodied selfhood/sainthood', *Australian Cultural History* (Special Issue on Bodies), 13, 1994, pp. 82–99, and 'Beyond Giddens: differentiating bodies', *Annual Review of Health Social Sciences* (Special Issue on Embodiment), 4, 1994, pp. 92–103.

Nick J. Fox is Senior Lecturer in Sociology at the University of Sheffield. He is author of *The Social Meaning of Surgery* (Open University Press, 1992) and *Postmodernism, Sociology and Health* (Open University Press and University of Minnesota Press, 1993).

Denise Gastaldo is a postdoctoral fellow at the Faculté des Sciences Infirmières, Université de Montréal, Canada. She is editor of the book *Paulo Freire at the Institute* (Institute of Education, University of London, 1995).

Jennifer Harding is Senior Lecturer in Communications at London Guildhall University. Her main areas of research interest/activity and publication are/have been: theories of the body, feminist theory and critiques of medicine, sexuality, cultural history and ethnography. Her recent publications examine 'the sexed body' and 'the hormonal body'.

Deborah Lupton is Associate Professor in Cultural Studies and Cultural Policy at Charles Sturt University, Bathurst, Australia. Her latest publications include *The Imperative of Health: Public Health and the Regulated Body* (Sage, 1995) and *Food, the Body and the Self* (Sage, 1996).

David McCallum teaches Sociology and Social Policy at Victoria University of Technology, Melbourne, Australia. His publications include *The Social Production of Merit* (Falmer Press, 1990). He is currently writing another book on personality disorder and dangerousness.

Sarah Nettleton is Lecturer in Social Policy in the Department of Social Policy and Social Work at the University of York. She is the author of *The Sociology of Health and Illness* (Polity Press, 1995) and *Power, Pain and Dentistry* (Open University Press, 1992) and a co-editor of *The Sociology of Health Promotion: Critical Analyses of Consumption, Lifestyle and Risk* (Routledge, 1995).

Thomas Osborne is a Lecturer in Sociology at the University of Bristol.

Alan Petersen is Senior Lecturer in Sociology at Murdoch University, Western Australia.

Bryan S. Turner is a Professor in Sociology, Dean of Arts and founder of the Centre for the Body and Society at Deakin University, Geelong, Victoria, Australia. His current research interests are in two areas: the sociology of ageing and generations, and the sociology of citizenship (with special reference to voluntary associations, the welfare state and globalisation). He is the editor of *The Blackwell Companion to Social Theory* (1996). With Mike Featherstone, he is the founding editor of the journal *Body and Society*.

Deborah Tyler teaches Sociology and Social Policy at the Footscray campus of Victoria University of Technology, Footscray, Victoria, Australia. She is the co-editor, with Denise Meredyth, of *Child and Citizen: Genealogies of Schooling and Subjectivity* (Institute for Cultural Policy Studies, Griffith University, 1993).

From governmentality to risk
Some reflections on Foucault's contribution to medical sociology

Bryan S. Turner

INTRODUCTION

During much of the post-war period, medical sociology lacked any significant theoretical direction or focus; it was an applied area of sociology, the aim of which was to assist general and community medicine in achieving greater patient compliance. This introductory observation on the recent history of medical sociology should, however, be qualified by noting two important and interrelated intellectual developments. The first is the general impact of Michel Foucault's analysis of power/knowledge which has come to influence a range of research topics and perspectives in the study of mental health and sickness since the publication in English of *Madness and Civilization* (Foucault 1965). The second crucial development, which is closely related to an interest in Foucault's social philosophy, is the tentative emergence of the sociology of the body as an analytical underpinning for medical sociology.

These two developments – the impact of Foucault on social science generally and the rise of the sociology of the body – pushed the discipline away from medical sociology towards the sociology of health and illness, that is towards a critical epistemology of disease categories as elements of the moral control of individuals and populations. This movement was based on an implicit slogan, namely that the body is historical. In this Foreword I want to comment on these contemporary developments in sociology as a framework for evaluating Foucault and as a perspective for the continuing growth of sociology. In particular, this Foreword attempts a comparison between Foucault's analysis of power/knowledge/discipline (namely 'governmentality') and Ulrich Beck's notion of 'risk society' (1992). These two frameworks are analysed as paradigms for understanding the new epidemiology of disease in late modern or postmodern society, but the philosophical choice between these two paradigms also indicates real tensions in contemporary society between the deregulation of the macro-global level (so-called 'risk society') and the micro-local requirement for a continuing micro-politics of surveillance and control (so-called 'carceral society').

SITUATING FOUCAULT: THE THEORY OF POWER

Foucault's academic reception within the English-speaking world was initially based upon his work on the history of psychiatry and the problem of madness in Western civilisation. Because Foucault was clearly associated politically with the interests of minority groups such as the mentally ill, prisoners and homosexuals, his contribution to sociology was seen in over-simple terms as a contribution to the study of social control. Foucault's critical work of psychiatry appeared in the context of the anti-psychiatry movement. Shortly after the English publication of *Madness and Civilization*, Thomas Szasz (1971) published *The Manufacture of Madness*. R.D. Laing's important *Sanity, Madness and the Family* had been published in 1964. In sociology (especially in North America) the dominant paradigm of deviance and mental illness was labelling theory which depended heavily on the work of H. Becker in *Outsiders* (1963). The intellectual and political context within which Foucault's work was launched guaranteed that his original philosophical and historical studies were interpreted as a contribution to social control theory, within which the mentally ill were a socially deviant group who challenged the basic norms and values of society, and who, as a consequence of being labelled deviant, were forced into careers of secondary deviance. In this context, Foucault's studies of normalisation through medical discourse had some relationship to Talcott Parsons's concept of 'the sick role' which interpreted sickness as the legitimisation of social deviance in which not being at work meant being deviant. The sick role normalised this absence from work and other functionally important roles (Holton and Turner 1986).

This interpretation of Foucault was reinforced by the appearance in English translations of *The Birth of the Clinic* (1973) and *Discipline and Punish* (1977). The complexity of Foucault's interest in 'technologies of the self' (Martin *et al.* 1988) only became apparent with the publication of the six-volume study of sexuality in the 1980s. Indeed the subtle interrelationships between Foucault's notion of the self and discipline were not adequately recognised until the importance of his treatment of 'governmentality' (Foucault 1991) was embraced within the secondary literature. Foucault was of course interested in the issue of social control, but this interest has to be situated within his theory of power, where governmentality can be seen as the bridge between the early historical interest in regimes of discipline and the later work on the production of the self, which began with his investigations into the ancient world and early Christianity. This intellectual interpretation is now fully supported by the biographical studies of Foucault's life and work by Didier Eribon (1992) and David Macey (1993). In retrospect, the single most important thread or theme in Foucault's diverse and complex work is the study of power (Simons 1995).

It is now clear that Foucault made three major contributions to contemporary social science, namely an analysis of power/knowledge, a contribution to the understanding of the emergence of the modern self through disciplinary technologies, and an analysis of governmentality, which integrated these dimensions into a single theory of power. Partly for the sake of economy of presentation and interpretation, I shall leave to one side Foucault's work on the philosophy of social science and methodology (Foucault 1970), recognising that in a more elaborate presentation of his work it would in fact be difficult to separate these dimensions of his research.

Foucault's analysis of power has been particularly useful in understanding the functions of the medical profession and the related spheres of psychiatry. Foucault has been important in locating, for example, the historical functions of the clinic as a site of bio-power (Foucault 1973). Foucault's theory of power can be seen as a critical reaction against both French Marxism and the existentialism of Sartre. Recent biographies (Eribon 1992) of Foucault have shown that his preoccupation with his own sexuality, his critique of Marxism and his involvement in the politics of the French academy did much to shape his theory of power. Foucault attempted to challenge the Marxist conceptualisation of power as a macro-structure such as the state which functioned to support industrial capitalism and which was displayed through major public institutions such as the police, the law and the church. Such a view of power was central to the work of Louis Althusser who was the dominant Marxist theoretician of the state and the ideological state apparatus in the 1960s.

By contrast, Foucault saw power as a relationship which was localised, dispersed, diffused and typically disguised through the social system, operating at a micro, local and covert level through sets of specific practices. Power is embodied in the day-to-day practices of the medical profession within the clinic, through the activities of social workers, through the mundane decision-making of legal officers, and through the religious practices of the church as they operate through such rituals as the confessional. This approach to politics had a particular message for radical Marxism, namely that the attempt to seize the state through political action would not destroy power, because power is rather like a colour dye diffused through the entire social structure and is embedded in daily practices. This view of power is very closely associated with Foucault's fascination with discipline, namely that power exists through the disciplinary practices which produce particular individuals, institutions and cultural arrangements. The disciplinary management of society results in a carceral society, that is a form of society in which the principles of Bentham's Panopticon are institutionalised through everyday routines and mundane arrangements.

Foucault's originality as a theorist and historian was to see how the ethical systems of ancient civilisations and early Christianity produced the self through practices of self-subjection. These ethical systems involved the identification of an ethical substance (such as desire) which is to be shaped through moral activity. Second, it requires subjection in which moral obligation is recognised (to subject oneself to God, for example). This subjection leads to the objectification of moral obligations into codes or discourses of ethics, such as the discourses of sexuality which Foucault studied under the notions of the 'care of the self' (Foucault 1986) and the 'use of pleasure' (Foucault 1985). These discourses of subjectivity then produce identities or roles such as the hysterical woman or the masturbatory child, and it is these identities which then become the object and focus of medicalisation and normalisation. In the modern period, the medicalisation of the menopausal woman in North America and the export of those discourses and identities to other societies such as Japan are clear illustrations of these processes (Lock 1993). These practices of subjection and self-formation also involve the emergence of complex pedagogies of self-transformation and education. The medieval confessional has now been elaborated and refined by modern forms of 'talking therapy' in psychoanalysis and, at another level of society, manuals of self-help (Giddens 1992). Finally, subjection requires the production of a moral order and an ethical ethos which becomes the organising principle of practices of the self; a moral code evolves by which moral identities are shaped and guided. In contemporary society, these goals typically include not only the ideology of self-fulfilment through self-knowledge, but a range of preventive health policies and measures which can be seen as an extension of these self-regulatory activities.

These ideas about power were further elaborated through Foucault's interest in 'governmentality', a system of power which articulated the triangular relationship between sovereignty, discipline and government. Governmentality (Foucault 1991), which emerged in the eighteenth century, is a mechanism for regulating and controlling populations through an apparatus of security. This governmental apparatus required a whole series of specific *savoirs* and was the foundation for the rise of the administrative state (Gutting 1989). A further important feature of Foucault's work was the analysis of the relationship between power and knowledge. Whereas liberal theory tended to separate power and knowledge on the grounds that truth is always corrupted by the exercise of power, Foucault saw that power and knowledge were always inevitably and inextricably interconnected so that any extension of power involved an increase in knowledge and every elaboration of knowledge involved an increase in power. Foucault approached this question typically through a consideration of populations and bodies. For example, the growth of penology and criminology was closely associated with the development of panoptic principles of surveillance and control. In a similar fashion the whole development of psychology and psychiatry was seen in terms of forms of knowledge, related to an extension of power over the subordinate populations of urban Europe. Foucault normally spoke about knowledge in the plural (*savoirs*) in order to illustrate the notion that specific forms of power required highly specific and detailed formations of knowledge.

This conceptual apparatus, which Foucault built up around the study of the history of ideas, the analysis of power and the explication of forms of discipline, proved enormously useful and important for medical sociologists in their attempt to understand the forms of power assumed by medical practices. Foucault's work permitted sociologists to think about the medicalisation of society within a new framework, where the exercise of medical power was seen in terms of local diffuse practices. The influence of Foucault is particularly significant in such publications as *Political Anatomy of the Body* (Armstrong 1983) *Medical Power and Social Knowledge* (Turner 1995), and *The Imperative of Health* (Lupton 1995). The medical sociology which was inspired by Foucault is typically understood to have made a distinctive break with the past. It was heavily informed by theoretical and philosophical analysis; it was highly critical of established medicine, seeking to provide alternative ways of examining mental illness and disease; it placed power and knowledge at the centre of the sociological understanding of medical institutions; and it showed how medical ideas of the moral character of disease operated at an everyday level.

As Foucault's work evolved and as more of Foucault's studies were translated into English, such as *The Use of Pleasure* (Foucault 1985) and *The Care of the Self* (Foucault 1986), it also became clear that for Foucault the study of medicine was part of a larger programme which examined the evolution of sexuality in European societies from classical Greece and how that evolution was intimately bound up with the transformation of medicine. In his final publications Foucault appeared to turn more and more to an analysis of the self in the context of medical history and the development of sexuality. His interest in how the self in Western societies was an effect of discourse of the self became increasingly obvious in his studies of 'technologies of the self' (Martin *et al.* 1988). Medical sociology and the sociology of health and illness were now seen to be both far broader in their terms of reference and also more central to the mainstream concerns of sociology as a whole.

Foucault provided a description of what one might call 'the institutions of normative coercion', such as the law, religion and medicine (Turner 1992). These institutions are coercive in the sense that they discipline individuals and exercise forms of surveillance over everyday life in such a way that actions are both produced and constrained by them. However, such institutions as the medical clinic are not coercive in the violent or authoritarian sense because they are readily accepted as legitimate and normative at the everyday level. These institutions of normative coercion exercise a moral authority over the individual by explaining individual 'problems' and providing solutions for them. In this sense we could say that medicine and religion exercise a hegemonic authority because their coercive character is often disguised and masked by their normative involvement in the troubles and problems of individuals. They are coercive, normative and also voluntary.

FOUCAULT AND THE SOCIOLOGY OF THE BODY

Although there was significant change in the intellectual evolution of Foucault's social philosophy, it is also clear that the body and populations played a continuous role in the analytic structure of his work. The body was the focus of military discipline, but it was also subject to the monastic regulation of medieval Catholicism. The body is the target of the medical gaze and governmentality. Generally speaking, health is a form of policing which is specifically concerned with the quality of the labour force. This view was clearly expressed by Foucault (1980a) in an article on 'The politics of health in the eighteenth century', where he suggested that the transformation of population:

> arguably concerns the economic-political effects of the accumula-
> tion of men. The great eighteenth-century demographic upswing in
> Western Europe, the necessity for co-ordinating and integrating it
> into the apparatus of production and the urgency of controlling it
> with finer and more adequate power mechanisms caused 'popula-
> tion', with its numerical variables of space and chronology,
> longevity and health, to emerge not only as a problem but as an
> object of surveillance, analysis, intervention, modification, etc.
>
> (Foucault 1980a: 171)

The nexus of knowledge/power was thus initially an effect of demographic changes, particularly the pressure of populations on systems of government and regulation from the eighteenth century. I have taken this demographic transformation to be, in fact, the major societal context for the emergence of modern forms of management, discipline and government (Turner 1987, 1992). It is the principal context for governmentality, as a regime which links self-subjection with societal regulation.

The body was clearly of major significance in *Discipline and Punish* but it also continued to play a crucial role in the larger project of *The History of Sexuality*, where Foucault was concerned with the body in relation to medicine and the body in relation to the development of the self within a Christian paradigm. Briefly, Foucault was interested in the production of bodies, the regulation of bodies and the representation of bodies within a context of disciplinary surveillance (Turner 1984). The integration of legal and medical controls over the body and identity was a theme in the study of hermaphrodites in *Herculine Barbin* (Foucault 1980b). Foucault's work on the production of sexual identity played a major part subsequently in the historical analysis of gender and sexuality (Laqueur 1990) and in the relationship between women and medicine (Martin 1987). In subsequent years the sociology of the body emerged as a major theme in medical sociology because it provided a powerful perspective on the socially constructed nature of disease

xvi   Bryan S. Turner

categories and the role of medicine in regulating individuals through regulating their bodies, and contributed also to new perspectives on the question of sexuality and medicine. Having been neglected as a theoretical topic for many decades the question of the human body has recently become a critical issue in the social sciences. There have been a number of major publications in this area resulting eventually in a new sub-field of sociology (Featherstone *et al.* 1991; Leder 1990; O'Neill 1989; Shilling 1993; Synnott 1993).

The causes and nature of this interest in the cultural aspects of the human body are both divergent and complex. However this new interest in the body is clearly related to the growing problems of human identity brought about by legal and social changes which in turn are a consequence of technical transformations in medicine, specifically in the area of human reproduction. There is also widespread public anxiety about the nature of contemporary epidemics such as HIV and AIDS which have drawn attention to the complexities of sexuality in modern society. These medical changes are also related to various social movements in modern society which seek to change social attitudes towards the body, particularly the gay and feminist move-ments. These anxieties about the body are also part of a broader concern about the demographic revolution of the last century, the process of ageing and the ecological deterioration of the environment. Within the context of capitalism, the body has also emerged as a significant feature in consumption advertising and consumer culture (Falk 1994). Cultural postmodernisation has also underlined the idea that the human body is simply a fabric or social product which has no ontological fixity. These postmodern questions about the body have brought a number of writers to speculate about the interaction between information systems, computer technology and the body.

Through these studies of the self, discipline and the body, medical sociology evolved more fully and effectively into the sociology of health and illness. At the same time, it became part of the mainstream interest of sociology, because the sociological study of health was perceived more openly as a sophisticated contribution to the study of power, where micro-practices of power were interpreted from Foucault's perspective of governmentality. These changes in the intellectual climate of the social sciences were direct consequences of the adoption of Foucault's perspective on bio-politics.

RISK SOCIETY AND CONTEMPORARY POLITICS: EVALUATING FOUCAULT

I have argued that to see Foucault's work as a contribution to the sociology of social control and deviance is, if not mistaken, at least a distorting over-simplification. Nevertheless, Foucault's focus on discipline, power and governmentality does have an intellectual proximity to Max Weber's study of instrumental rationality and bureaucracy, and to Theodor Adorno's contributions to the notion of an administered society. It also suggests a parallel to Erving Goffman's notion of the total institution. The carceral society indicates a regime of micro-regulations and disciplines which operate through a complex web of self-subjection. In short, we can see Foucault as part of a sociological tradition which emphasises the importance of regulation and administration as key features of 'modern society'. Like Weber, Foucault provided a profound insight into the bureaucratic mentality of a society dominated by the logic of instrumental rationality. How relevant then is Foucault to a social environment which is seen to be postmodern, deregulated and risky?

Throughout the 1980s there were major changes in the structure of the economy and government, which in retrospect we can see as part of the Thatcherite revolution in the marketisation of social relations, including the marketisation of the provision of social services. Managerialism, privatisation and deregulation were dimensions of a profound globalisation of the world economy the effects of which were particularly visible in the areas of the service industries, tourism, consumerism and labour markets. We can see the current enthusiasm for the concept of 'risk society' as a response to this general sense that the modern world has become more uncertain, contingent, flexible and risky. It appears to be in structure and ethos very far removed from the carceral society with its dependable and recognisable processes and procedures.

In the health field these changes have been profound. The traditions of centralised mechanisms for the provision of social security and welfare have been replaced by a logic of internal markets, competitive tendering and devolved budgets. The very notion of 'security' sits oddly with the contemporary enthusiasm for a discourse of entrepreneurish, just-in-time management systems and the culture of risk. These changes in bureaucratic structures have occurred alongside major epidemiological changes which in a sinister fashion appear to mimic the contingency of the market place; namely the spread of AIDs and other infectious diseases, the deterioration of the food supply, the danger of inter-species disease such as 'mad cow disease' and the associated risks of Creuzfeldt Jacob's disease. These changes are not easily encapsulated within Foucault's language of discipline and control. It is true that Foucault was aware of changes in the provision of welfare (Foucault 1988) and it is also the case that his notion of governmentality can be extended to analyse some aspects of a risk environment. However, there is a profound tension between the metaphors which lie behind risk society and governmentality (Turner 1995: 218–27).

How might we, at least in theoretical terms, resolve some of these tensions? There are a number of possibilities (Turner 1994: 167–82). To some extent we might argue that financial deregulation in the 1980s produced a global environment of political and economic uncertainty between nation states but within each industrial society the need for micro-surveillance and discipline continued with greater intensity; indeed the importance of a carceral society has increased with the growth of externalised macro-risk. As the global economy develops into a culture of risk, the nation state is forced to invest more and more in internal systems of governmentality. Second, a risk society, based on deregulation and devolution, often requires more subtle and systematic forms of control. For example, the state is forced to create regulatory systems of quality control where public utilities have been privatised. Third, financial deregulation increases the scale of economic risk. Where major companies and public institutions fall into debt and bankruptcy, governments typically intervene, despite their ideological commitment to privatisation and deregulation, to save such institutions. Fourth, we can in fact argue that modern societies are structured by two apparently contradictory processes: the growth of risk cultures and the McDonaldisation of society (Ritzer 1993). McDonaldisation is the application of Fordist production methods and rational managerialism to the fast-food industry which is then extended to all sectors of society. McDonaldisation reduces uncertainty and unpredictability; it is, in short, a response to risk and uncertainty. McDonaldisation removes surprises from everyday life by an extension of instrumental rationality to production, distribution and consumption. After the McDonaldisation of the fast-food industry, these principles have also been applied to universities and medicine. McDentists and McDoctors extend the principles of cheapness, standardisation and reliability to the health industry. The welfare and health system is now a complex mixture of risk culture and McDonaldisation of services. Finally, the notion of generalised risk in the environment may lead to greater surveillance and control through the promotion of preventive medicine (Lupton 1995). The AIDs 'epidemic' creates a political climate within which intervention and control are seen to be both necessary and benign. Individuals need, especially in the area of sexual etiquette, to become self-regulating and self-forming.

If Foucault's theories of sexuality and governmentality are to continue to inspire and to shape the future development of the sociology of health and illness, followers of Foucault will be compelled to address the new environment of risk cultures, political contingencies and deregulated welfare systems. The burden of dependency, with the ageing of Western societies, is being answered increasingly with the privatisation of medicine and a doctrine of obligation. The traditional notions of citizen rights (to health and social welfare) are being questioned by a liberal ideology of individual obligation (to save and to create personal bases of security). The problem of mental health in society is being resolved, not with greater surveillance, but with de-institutionalisation. In America, the number of residents in state mental hospitals fell from 513,000 in 1950 to 111,000 in 1986 as a consequence of a policy of de-institutionalisation. The economic cost of state intervention in health care has in most advanced societies resulted in new policies of privatisation, 'out-sourcing', 'down-sizing', internal markets, managerialism and de-institutionalisation. Such economic and social processes are not easily described or explained within Foucault's paradigm of the disciplinary society, panopticism and governmentality. The intellectual challenge is to comprehend the structures and institutions of postmodern society within the conceptual apparatus of Foucault's understanding of governmentality.

REFERENCES

Armstrong, D. (1983) *Political Anatomy of the Body. Medical Knowledge in Britain in the Twentieth Century*, Cambridge: Cambridge University Press.

Beck, U. (1992) *Risk Society: Towards a New Modernity*, London: Sage.

Becker, H.S. (1963) *Outsiders. Studies in the Sociology of Deviance*, New York: Free Press.

Eribon, D. (1992) *Michel Foucault*, London: Faber and Faber.

Falk, P. (1994) *The Consuming Body*, London: Sage.

Featherstone, M., Hepworth, M. and Turner, B.S. (eds) (1991) *The Body. Social Process and Cultural Theory*, London: Sage.

Foucault, M. (1965) *Madness and Civilization. The History of Insanity in the Age of Reason*, New York: Random House.

Foucault, M. (1970) *The Order of Things*, London: Tavistock.

Foucault, M. (1973) *The Birth of the Clinic. An Archaeology of Medical Perception*, London: Tavistock.

Foucault, M. (1977) *Discipline and Punish. The Birth of the Prison*, London: Allen Lane.

Foucault, M. (1980a) 'The politics of health in the eighteenth century', in C. Gordon (ed.) *Power/Knowledge. Selected Interviews and Other Writings, 1972–1977*, Brighton: The Harvester Press, pp. 166–82.

Foucault, M. (1980b) *Herculine Barbin. Being the Recently Discovered Memoirs of a Nineteenth-Century French Hermaphrodite*, Brighton: The Harvester Press.

Foucault, M. (1985) *The History of Sexuality, Volume 2: The Use of Pleasure*, New York: Random House.

Foucault, M. (1986) *The History of Sexuality, Volume 3: The Care of the Self*, New York: Random House.

Foucault, M. (1988) 'Social security', in L.D. Kritzman (ed.) *Michel Foucault. Politics Philosophy Culture, Interviews and Other Writings, 1977–1984*, New York and London: Routledge, pp. 159–77.

Foucault, M. (1991) 'Governmentality', in G. Burchell, C. Gordon and P. Miller (eds) *The Foucault Effect*, Brighton: Harvester Wheatsheaf, pp. 87–194.

Giddens, A. (1992) *The Transformation of Intimacy. Sexuality, Love and Eroticism in Modern Societies*, Cambridge: Polity Press.

Gutting, G. (1989) *Michel Foucault's Archaeology of Scientific Reason*, Cambridge: Cambridge University Press.

Holton, R.J. and Turner, B.S. (1986) *Talcott Parsons on Economy and Society*, London and New York: Routledge and Kegan Paul.

Laing, R.D. (1964) *Sanity, Madness and the Family, Volume 1: Families of Schizophrenics*, London: Tavistock.

Laqueur, T. (1990) *Making Sex. Body and Gender from the Greeks to Freud*, Cambridge, Massachusetts: Harvard University Press.

Leder, D. (1990) *The Absent Body*, Chicago and London: Chicago University Press.

Lock, M. (1993) *Encounters with Aging. Mythologies of Menopause in Japan and North America*, Berkeley and Los Angeles: University of California Press.

Lupton, D. (1995) *The Imperative of Health. Public Health and the Regulated Body*, London: Sage.

Macey, D. (1993) *The Lives of Michel Foucault*, London: Hutchinson.

Martin, E. (1987) *The Woman in the Body: A Cultural Analysis of Reproduction*, Milton Keynes: Open University Press.

Martin, L.H., Gutman, H. and Hutton, P.H. (eds) (1988) *Technologies of the Self. A Seminar with Michel Foucault*, London: Tavistock.

O'Neill, J. (1989) *The Communicative Body. Studies in Communicative Philosophy, Politics and Sociology*, Evanston, Illinois: Northwestern University Press.

Ritzer, G. (1993) *The McDonaldization of Society*, Thousand Oaks, California: Pine Forge Press.

Shilling, C. (1993) *The Body and Social Theory*, London: Sage.

Simons, J. (1995) *Foucault and the Political*, London: Routledge.

Synnott, A. (1993) *The Body Social. Symbolism, Self and Society*, London and New York: Routledge.

Szasz, T.S. (1971) *The Manufacture of Madness. A Comparative Study of the Inquisition and the Mental Health Movement*, London: Routledge and Kegan Paul.

Turner, B.S. (1984) *The Body and Society. Explorations in Social Theory*, Oxford: Blackwell.

Turner, B.S. (1987) 'The rationalisation of the body. Reflections on modernity and discipline', in S. Lash and S. Whimster (eds) *Max Weber, Rationality and Modernity*, London: Allen and Unwin, pp. 222–41.

Turner, B.S. (1992) *Regulating Bodies. Essays in Medical Sociology*, London and New York: Routledge.

Turner, B.S. (1994) *Orientalism, Postmodernism and Globalism*, London: Routledge.

Turner, B.S. (1995) *Medical Power and Social Knowledge*, revised edition, London: Sage.

Acknowledgements

The editors would like to thank all the contributors for agreeing to be part of this project, and for their enthusiasm. They would also like to thank Heather Gibson and Fiona Bailey from Routledge for their support and editorial assistance. Alan Petersen is grateful to Murdoch University, which granted him a period of study leave in 1995 and paid for his travel to the UK which allowed him to make contact with a number of the contributors, and to his colleagues in the Sociology Program for providing intellectual stimulation. He would also like to thank Ros Porter, who has accompanied him on his travels and sustained his work in innumerable ways. Robin Bunton would like to thank colleagues and friends in the School of Human Studies, University of Teesside, especially Mike Featherstone, Barbara Cox and Roy Boyne. Special thanks to Lesley Jones for supporting the project and for reading through early parts of the text. Thanks also to Sue Jackson.

Introduction

Foucault's medicine

Robin Bunton and Alan Petersen

The reception of Foucault's work in the social sciences and humanities has been truly phenomenal. It is difficult to overestimate his influence over the last decade or so. Few subject areas remain untouched by his analyses of discourse, power and governance. A burgeoning 'Foucault industry' has produced books and articles exploring the implications of these concepts for social and political theory as whole, and for studies of government, body regulation and sexuality and gender. The study of health and medicine is no exception and his influence is so profound here that we cannot think of a great many topics without some reliance on his work. Foucault's approach has opened up new lines of enquiry, crossed disciplinary boundaries and made links between areas that have hitherto been treated as discrete, such as the merging of pathological anatomy and health policy, and sexuality and bio-medical practice. Foucault deserves our attention if no other reason than that health and medicine were major themes in his enquiries and were used to illustrate his broader theories about the relationship between power and knowledge (see Foucault 1965, 1975, 1980, 1991). It would be wrong, however, to see Foucault's contribution to the study of health and medicine as limited to his own substantive enquiries. Foucault's legacy is best assessed in the light of the influence of his work on subsequent thinking and research. There has been a noticeable 'Foucault effect' in the study of health and medicine as elsewhere (Burchell *et al.* 1991). In planning this book, we sought to convey something of the breadth of recent Foucauldian scholarship in the area of health and medicine, while recognising that we could never do justice to the broad range of work that is being undertaken.

Most of the authors of the following chapters are known for their research in the sociology of health and medicine, though their interests clearly extend beyond the discipline of sociology. This work illustrates how researchers are currently engaging with Foucault's work and the problematisations of health he developed. In turn, their work problematises and critiques Foucault's work itself. There is a necessary reflexivity in this exercise. Foucault, as Kate Soper (1995) observes, makes those who problematise his thought acutely conscious of the pieties they bring to it. We are well aware, since his death, of the packaging of Foucault's thought and the dangers in providing too limited a reading of it and that at times it is difficult to distinguish between what Foucault wrote and what has been represented as his ideas. We are also aware that with Foucault, as with Marx and Nietzsche, the point is not simply to interpret his work but 'to use it' (Rajchman 1995). This collection attempts to bring together some of those who are currently using Foucault to study health and medicine. They necessarily draw upon and give different readings of Foucault's work but, with a similar exploratory line of enquiry, they attempt to produce varying problematisations of contemporary health and medicine. Foucault's work encourages new approaches to old problems and, as David McCallum (in chapter 3) so eloquently puts it, 'rather than providing "schemas" and closures, the implied intellectual invitation is to take up his methods of enquiry as a way of charting new territories and formulating questions in different sorts of ways'.

These papers focus upon some familiar health topics such as madness, child health, health policy and health education, though the approach taken is distinct from that of, say, the sociology of health and illness. The collection also addresses newer sites of health care, including eating disorders, hormone replacement, risk management, self-care and consumption. These areas are representative of a changing world of health. As Bryan Turner notes above, if Foucault's theories are to continue to inspire, then analysts will be compelled to address new environments of risk cultures, political contingencies and deregulated health and welfare systems. These papers illustrate how Foucauldian studies of health and medicine are exploring recent changes in health and health care. Some familiar Foucauldian topics emerge throughout the chapters, in particular the discourses of health and disease, the body and the self, and governmentality. These topics broadly correspond to some of the changing focuses of Foucault's work throughout his life (McHoul and Grace 1993). We use them here for heuristic purposes where they serve to roughly divide up the contributions into three of the four parts of this volume. For the moment, these categories are pivotal in Foucauldian studies of health. They are far from being definitive and we would expect them, in turn, to be re-problematised.

In Part I, concerned with the problematisation of Foucault's work itself, David Armstrong's and Nick Fox's chapters implicitly question this scheme. By drawing attention to the range of topics and the different readings (or '*differends*') of Foucault, both authors remind us of our continuing fabrication of Foucauldian method. These critical pieces serve to introduce the collection as a whole, as a set of treatments of Foucault and health and medicine. In chapter 1, David Armstrong alerts us to Foucault's problematisation of the author and identifies some of the 'Foucaults' that have been evident in the sociology of health and illness. Armstrong's chapter outlines the influence of four of Foucault's books which have had, and continue to have, an effect: *Madness and Civilization, Birth of the Clinic, Discipline and Punish* and *The History of Sexuality, Volume 1*. By reading the different readings of Foucault, Armstrong usefully charts Foucault's influence on writers and areas of study. In chapter 2, Nick Fox argues that Foucault's ontology is ambiguous and contradictory and proposes alternative sources for exploring, theorising and researching discourse, the body and the self. He suggests that the use of texts and framing derived from the writing of Barthes, Derrida and Lyotard offers useful points of departure. Lyotard's notion of the *differend* is used to illustrate how we may more sucessfully account for intertextuality and the play of difference and resistance. Both the above chapters are useful starting points, reminding us of the ways in which this volume engages with Foucault's incomplete ontology.

Part II deals with one of the significant legacies of Foucault's work – the concept of discourse – which was employed extensively in his analysis of the subject. For Foucault, the subject is constituted through discourse rather than having a prediscursive existence. As he himself indicated towards the end of his life, his objective in his work had been to 'create a history of the different modes by which, in our culture, human beings are made subjects' (1982: 208). In his later writings on the history of sexuality he began to focus on those practices through which human beings turned themselves into subjects (Foucault 1985, 1986). Foucault's corpus concentrated on the modern period and he sought to challenge the modernist assumption of historical progression, continuity and unilinear development – a narrative which serves to confirm rather than challenge the beliefs and practices of the present. His method of genealogy or 'history of the present' directs attention to discontinuities and ruptures in thought and involves recognition of multiple determinations and the role of chance. It is a method that has an explicit theoretical and political goal: to disrupt the taken-for-grantedness of the present and to show how things could be different. As Deborah Tyler notes below, it is not an attempt to understand the past from the point of view of the present, but rather to disturb the self-evident present with the past. This method has proved a powerful tool of deconstruction, as is evident from a long line of studies in the social sciences. Foucault's genealogical approach to sexuality has, for example, helped stimulate the development of a rich field of historical enquiry into the social construction of sex and sexuality (Hausman 1995; Katz 1995; Laqueur 1990; Weeks 1985). Historical research such as this, by pointing to shifts in discursive practices, indicates the inherent instability of the present, and allows us to imagine things being otherwise.

In different ways David McCallum's and Deborah Tyler's chapters demonstrate the emergence of certain subjectivities in the discourses on mental health and criminality, and on child development, respectively. In chapter 3, McCallum disturbs the certainties and truths of the categories of personality and personality disorder by providing a genealogical analysis of the conceptual terrain of the problem of the 'dangerous individual'. Rather than accepting accounts of an ahistorical problem individual, the categories of the present can be understood as the combination of a number of elements. On the one hand there developed an increased individualisation of the population in the late nineteenth century, accomplished through a range of statistical procedures, administrative reforms and social hygiene strategies. These developments were coupled with a twentieth-century growth in the 'psy-disciplines' which sought to understand the internal workings of the individual, and increasing attempts to regulate citizens through the advancement of norms of personal life. Knowledge of the person is made possible by means of a complexity of interrelations between law, psychiatry and the institutional spaces in which they operate.

In chapter 4, Tyler examines and disturbs a similar scientific 'discovery' – the propensity of boys to display 'bad habits' more than girls. She examines the conditions of possibility that allowed boys' and girls' behaviours to become 'recognised' as 'at risk' or 'maladjusted' at all. She accounts for the techniques of governing the child and the strategies for modifying the behaviour in the kindergarten and other educational milieux. The contemporary Australian Temperament Project casts boys as an 'at risk population'. This is due not to 'discoveries' of the inner working of the human mind but to the techniques of governing child populations developed throughout the early part of this century. For this discourse it would appear that what is known about the soul of the child is less important than what is known about what can be done to deal with it.

The issue of discursive domination is examined critically by Deborah Lupton in chapter 5. Lupton compares the similarities and differences between the orthodox medicalisation critique and Foucauldian commentaries on bio-medicine. She notes that whereas supporters of the 'medicalisation' critique see power as being primarily repressive, Foucauldian commentators acknowledge the productive aspects of disciplinary power in the 'clinical gaze'. However, as Lupton points out, both orthodox sociological accounts of medical knowledge and Foucauldian accounts tend to ignore a number of features of the medical encounter – such as the unconscious and the emotions – which are in need of further exploration.

Part III turns to the analysis of the body and of the self, and of their relationship. As Turner indicates above, the body was of major significance in Foucault's work, and his unique perspective on the body as a focus for disciplinary power has undoubtedly helped to recast thinking about the nature of the body and about the operations of power in modern societies. The analysis of 'bio-power' gives us two axes through which power works in relation to the human body: one working on the individual body, the so called 'anatomo-politics of the body', the other as a 'bio-politics of population' working through population. Such an approach to the body was to have a significant reordering effect on the sociology of health and illness (Petersen 1993; Turner 1995). Foucault conceives the body not as natural or neutral but as reproduced in specific sets of practices and discourse. His approach draws attention to the techniques used for managing populations or the social body, and particularly the 'apparatus of normalisation' (Armstrong 1983: 51). In *The Birth of the Clinic* (1975), for instance, he showed how, during the nineteenth century, there emerged a unique discourse of 'the body' which shaped the way it was seen, described and acted upon. Increasingly the body was objectified and subject to new techniques of power – disciplinary power. Medicine played a key role in the new perception of 'the body' through its focus on pathological anatomy where disease was located in the body of the patient. This discourse differed from that which had prevailed up until the end of the eighteenth century, when medicine related much more to health than to normality (1975: 35).

In chapter 6, Denise Gastaldo argues that health education has come to play an increasingly important role in the exercise of 'bio-power' through its association with illness prevention and health promotion.

Drawing on data from her study of health education policies and practices in the Brazilian national health system, Gastaldo describes how discourses on health education have contributed to the management of social and individual bodies by introducing new knowledge, surveillance and disciplinary techniques into everyday life. By inviting subjects to make decisions about their health and become actively involved in the care of themselves and their communities, health education invokes self-autonomy and self-governance. Like a number of other contributors to this collection, Gastaldo seeks to emphasise the complexity of modern relations of power which depend not upon the direct control of subjects through coercive means but rather upon creating a sphere for their regulated autonomy.

Foucault has been criticised for his inattention to gender in his own analyses of the body and the self (see e.g. Barrett 1991: 151–2; Flax 1990: 212). But his concepts have nevertheless been highly influential in feminism, both in terms of explorations of the utility of his concepts for feminist theory and practice and for the analysis of such areas as eating disorders, reproductive technologies, and the regulation of women through medical discourse and in health care settings (see e.g. Diamond and Quinby 1988; Hausman 1995; McNay 1992; Oudshoorn 1994; Ramazanoğlu 1993; Robertson 1992; Sawicki 1991). Foucault's work offers feminism a sophisticated perspective on the power relations of health and of medicine, and draws attention to the productive potential of medical knowledges and practices, and the opportunities this creates for resistance. For example, new reproductive medical technologies create such categories of individual as the infertile, surrogate and genetically impaired mothers, mothers whose bodies are not fit for pregnancy (either biologically or socially), mothers who are psychologically unfit for fertility treatments, mothers whose wombs are hostile environments to foetuses and so on. At the same time, the possibility of new sites of resistance is created, such as the case of single and lesbian women who challenge these norms by demanding access to infertility treatments (Sawicki 1991: 84). Foucault's work challenges those feminist perspectives which posit women as victims of a violent and repressive patriarchy. In the area of medical technologies, for example, it leads one to question why many women see new medical technologies as enabling and have at times been among the strongest proponents of their development and use. More fundamentally, however, Foucault's work problematises what has come to be taken as the stable object of most feminist analyses: the sexed body.

In her analysis of hormone replacement therapy (HRT), in chapter 7,

Jennifer Harding argues that feminist and medical discourses converge in their reference to an already sexed body. She compares medical and feminist discourse on HRT and their subject and audience – the post-menopausal woman – and examines how they both participate in the sexing of bodies. Feminist women's health discourse, like medical discourse, presupposes the existence of 'sex' as a fixed category and precondition for defining menopause and designating individuals as either requiring or not requiring treatment. The feminist critique fails to appreciate the extent to which bio-medicine provides the language through which bodies become culturally intelligible. Through their deployment of the construct of 'risk', both medical and feminist health discourses call upon women to make themselves objects of self-surveillance. One outcome of this is that ageing women's desires are circumscribed by a responsibility to resist their own 'decrepitude'. This chapter explores not just dominant techniques of the body and the self but also 'unofficial' or subjugated knowledges, though in this case both produce similar technologies of the self, thus underlining, as Foucault was so fond of doing, the ironies of the power effects of 'new social movement' politics.

In chapter 8, Liz Eckermann examines the relevance of Foucault's ideas to feminism through an analysis of embodiment and gendered subjectivities, with particular reference to self-starvation. As Eckermann points out, both in his early work on the body and in his later work on the self – as articulated in the last two volumes of *The History of Sexuality* – Foucault offers useful conceptual tools for sociologically understanding the body and those factors shaping the modern 'epidemic' of self-starvation. His concepts of surveillance and confession, for example, prove useful in the analysis of behavioural modification techniques used in treatment and of the self-disciplinary strategies brought into play in the attempt to achieve the ideal body appearance (e.g. weight reduction). As Eckermann concludes, Foucault's work is invaluable in developing a feminist political practice, for generating new research questions, and in providing suggestions for therapeutic intervention.

In Part IV, the chapters explore the application of Foucault's notion of governmentality to the analysis of health policy, health promotion and the consumption of health. Governmentality is an overarching concern that runs throughout all parts of the book, reflecting Foucault's rather broad notion of the concept, which he described as the contact point between technologies of domination (including discourse) and technologies of the self (Foucault 1988: 19). In chapter 9, Thomas

Osborne draws upon Foucault's (and Canguilhem's) work to break out of what he terms 'reactive' accounts of the relation between health and policy. Such accounts, he argues, tend to see health policy as a reaction to objective health needs, on the one hand, and state of health as the result of the effectiveness of health policy, on the other. The concept of governmentality directs attention to the problematisations of government, and to policy as a creative rather than as a reactive endeavour. Health is seen not as an absolute or determinate concept, but rather as a relative and indeterminate one – a by-product of governmental intervention. The discourses of health policy are examined from the point of view of liberal and neo-liberal rationalities of government, a theme that is taken up in the final three chapters.

Alan Petersen, Sarah Nettleton and Robin Bunton focus on the particular techniques of governance associated with the discourses of health promotion and 'care of the self' in these remaining chapters. Common themes explored are the salience of risk culture, the central role of expertise in liberal technologies of government, and the emergence of the concept of the enterprising self. Techniques for empowerment and participation are analysed as double-edged: extending the 'clinical gaze' whilst constructively managing the population. The reliance of neo- or advanced liberal societies on an enterprising, self-caring subject is a theme developed by Foucault in the latter part of his career. Although Foucault's historical approach is tied to a critique of the autonomous, rational, self-reflexive subject of Western liberal humanism, his later work acknowledges a self that is autonomous and able to extricate itself from normalising judgements and disciplinary practices. He left us with, as Schrift puts it:

> The task of thinking a notion of a subject that is both autonomous and disciplined, both actively self-forming and passively self-constructed, as he left us to think about the emergence of a modern state whose exercising of pastoral power both totalizes and individualizes.

(1995: 34)

The final chapters take up these problematics in different ways.

Alan Petersen, in chapter 10, identifies the central technology of newer approaches to health characteristic of health promotion and the new public health, that of risk management. The analysis of risk and health has been given renewed force in sociology of late through the work of Ulrich Beck (1992, 1995) and Anthony Giddens (1991). Petersen develops the implications of the analysis of risk for governance and the management of populations, drawing upon the work of Castel, who identified the shift in focus in contemporary health and social care from 'dangerousness' to 'risk'. This shift has had a profound influence on relationships between experts and subjects and requires more diverse intervention strategies. Risk appears here as a technology by which the freedom of the neo-liberal subject is generated. The rationality of neo-liberalism produces an entrepreneurial self, endowed with the ability to manage its own risks and risk behaviour. Health promotion is a strategy that engenders risk minimisation by attention to lifestyle and the privatisation of risk. 'Healthism' and 'bodyism' are integral processes.

This theme is also taken up by Sarah Nettleton in chapter 11 on governing the risky self. Referring to contemporary health policy and health promotion practice in the UK, she examines how current styles of governance produce autonomous, enterprising reflexive selves and communities who manage risks. This is not a one-way relationship of domination relying on certainties but the outcome of reciprocity between aggregate and individual actions. Power is exercised because subjects are able to react to expert knowledge. Like a number of other contributors (e.g. Lupton in chapter 5 and Gastaldo in chapter 6), she recognises the productive aspects of disciplinary power at work; in this case in health promotion discourse. Challenge to expert knowledge, she notes, is integral to this style of governance. Drawing upon Rose's (1992) analysis of governmentality in liberal democracies, this chapter points out that subjects are not simply subjected to policies and programmes but are required to participate.

In the final chapter, Robin Bunton analyses the technologies of governance associated with advanced liberalism through a study of changing representations of health and self-care in the *Good Housekeeping* magazine since 1959. Bunton notes a growth during this period in 'health-related' goods and services in line with the increasingly market-oriented approach to health and the emergence of the more discerning, health-conscious subject. Products have become increasingly marketed with an eye to their expressive as well as instrumental function; for what they signify about the identity of the consumer. This can be seen with the marketing of new 'soft' toilet tissue products, which represented a shift from a focus on the purely hygienic aspects of the product towards an emphasis on the luxuriousness of the product. At the same time, new, preventive, 'risk-oriented' knowledge was becoming more apparent while challenges to medical authority were becoming routine. It can be seen how also, during this period, 'psy' expertise was employed in governing acts of consumption: in establishing the psychological significance of products, and in their design and marketing. As this analysis illustrates, the health consumer of advanced liberalism is positioned not as a passive, cultural dope but as an active, enterprising and self-caring subject capable of selectively consuming health products and selectively reading his or her own health messages.

In collecting the chapters in this volume we are acutely aware of gaps and omissions, both in topics and in authors. We have not attempted to produce a collection representative of a field of study in this sense. Nor is it an attempt to identify or assess the gaps and missing topics in post-Foucauldian scholarship (such as phenomenological study, 'race' or a post-colonial focus). Rather we have brought together some critically appreciative papers illustrating the possibilities that Foucault's work continues to bring to the study of health and medicine. It shows how some researchers are drawing on Foucault's work to use and 'diagnose' the health and medicine of our times. In different ways these authors have sought to open up and problematise areas of study and have produced different readings of Foucault. They have drawn upon the 'toolbox' of Foucault's work and hopefully, in so doing, have made these tools more available to others.

REFERENCES

Armstrong, D. (1983) *Political Anatomy of the Body: Medical Knowledge in Britain in the Twentieth Century*, Cambridge: Cambridge University Press.

Barrett, M. (1991) *The Politics of Truth: From Marx to Foucault*, Cambridge: Polity Press.

Beck, U. (1992) *Risk Society: Towards a New Modernity*, London: Sage.

Beck, U. (1995) *Ecological Politics in an Age of Risk*, Cambridge: Polity Press.

Burchell, G., Gordon, C. and Miller, P. (eds) (1991) *The Foucault Effect: Studies in Governmentality*, Hemel Hempstead: Harvester Wheatsheaf.

Diamond, I. and Quinby, L. (eds) (1988) *Feminism and Foucault: Reflections on Resistance*, Boston: Northeastern University Press.

Flax, J. (1990) *Thinking Fragments: Psychoanalysis, Feminism and Post-modernism in the Contemporary West*, Berkeley: University of California Press.

Foucault, M. (1965) *Madness and Civilization*, trans. R. Howard, New York: Vintage.

Foucault, M. (1975) *The Birth of the Clinic: An Archaeology of Medical Perception*, New York: Vintage Books.

Foucault, M. (1980) *The History of Sexuality, Volume 1: An Introduction*, New York: Vintage Books.

Foucault, M. (1982) 'The subject and power' (Afterword), in H.L. Dreyfus and

P. Rabinow, *Michel Foucault: Beyond Structuralism and Hermeneutics*, Hemel Hempstead: Harvester Wheatsheaf.

Foucault, M. (1985) *The Use of Pleasure, The History of Sexuality, Volume 2*, London: Penguin.

Foucault, M. (1986) *The Care of the Self, The History of Sexuality, Volume 3*, London: Penguin.

Foucault, M. (1988) 'Technologies of the self', in L.H. Martin, H. Gutman and P. Hutton (eds) *Technologies of the Self: A Seminar with Michel Foucault*, London: Tavistock Publications.

Foucault, M. (1991) 'The politics of health in the eighteenth century', in P. Rabinow (ed.) *The Foucault Reader*, London: Penguin.

Giddens, A. (1991) *Modernity and Self-Identity: Self and Society in the Late Modern Age*, Cambridge: Polity Press.

Hausman, B. (1995) *Changing Sex: Transsexualism, Technology, and the Idea of Gender*, Durham, North Carolina: Duke University Press.

Katz, J. (1995) *The Invention of Heterosexuality*, New York: Penguin.

Laqueur, T. (1990) *Making Sex: Body and Gender from the Greeks to Freud*, Cambridge, Massachusetts: Harvard University Press.

McHoul, A. and Grace, W. (1993) *A Foucault Primer: Discourse, Power and the Subject*, London: University College London Press.

McNay, L. (1992) *Foucault and Feminism: Power, Gender and the Self*, Cambridge: Polity Press.

Oudshoorn, N. (1994) *Beyond the Natural Body: An Archaeology of Sex Hormones*, London: Routledge.

Petersen, A.R. (1993) 'Re-defining the subject? The influence of Foucault on the sociology of health and illness', in B.S. Turner, L. Eckermann, D. Colquhoun and P. Crotty (eds) *Annual Review of Health Social Science*, Volume 3, Geelong: Centre for the Study of the Body and Society, Deakin University.

Rajchman, J. (1995) 'Foucault ten years after', *New Formations*, 25: 214–20.

Ramazanoğlu, C. (ed.) (1993) *Up Against Foucault: Explorations of Some Tensions Between Foucault and Feminism*, London: Routledge.

Robertson, M. (1992) *Starving in the Silences: An Exploration of Anorexia Nervosa*, Sydney: Allen and Unwin.

Rose, N. (1992) 'Governing the enterprising self', in P. Heelas and P. Morris (eds) *The Values of the Enterprise Culture*, London: Routledge.

Sawicki, J. (1991) *Disciplining Foucault: Feminism, Power and the Body*, New York: Routledge.

Schrift, A.D. (1995) 'Reconfiguring the subject as a process of self: following Foucault's Nietzschean trajectory to Butler, Laclau/Mouffe, and beyond', *New Formations*, 25: 28–39.

Soper, D. (1995) 'Forget Foucault?', *New Formations*, 25: 21–7.

Turner, B.S. (1995) *Medical Power and Social Knowledge*, 2nd edn, London: Sage.

Weeks, J. (1985) *Sexuality and its Discontents: Meanings, Myths and Modern Sexualities*, London: Routledge and Kegan Paul.

Part I

Fabricating Foucault

Chapter 1

Foucault and the sociology of health and illness

A prismatic reading

David Armstrong

INTRODUCTION

Who is Foucault? I do not know, and I do not really care. I confess that I
have not read any of the biographies that have been written about him
and I have no interest in his personal life. Indeed, if, as in some
Shakespearean authorship mystery, I was told that he never¯really
existed and that the books bearing his name were written by a number
of different people it would not bother me. How then can I write about
an author who may or may not have existed?

In his essay 'What is an author?', Foucault identified a shift in the
'author function' over the centuries. In medieval times the truth of the
text was to be discovered in the truth of the author – a saint, being who
he was, only spoke the truth while heretics were known to write
untruths. But in modern times, that relationship has been reversed; the
truth of the author is to be found in the truth of the text as we scan the
author's words to find out who he or she really was. In other words, the
answer to the question 'Who is Foucault?' is given by whoever we infer
from the texts bearing his name. But of course there are many different
readings/inferences despite attempts to find the 'real Foucault' behind
them (and then in some medieval hegemonic gesture claim to grasp
what Foucault really did mean).

Many different readings and many different Foucaults. Mine can
only be one such reading: if others got it 'wrong' then that reflects no
more than my personal reading. This means that in the following review
of the influence of Foucault on the sociology of health and illness my
task is not to describe the links between the man and the sociological
researcher but to explore the connections between some texts that bear
his imprimatur and the reader.

Foucault was a prolific writer. Besides a number of books there were many essays and interviews. Trying to determine the supposed 'influence' of this corpus would be a massive task, even if it was a legitimate one. A more focused goal for this chapter is to identify some 'influences' of four main texts as evidenced by explicit acknowledgements (in the form of discussion or reference) in my own writings and those of others. This will involve reconstructing that engagement between text and reader as Foucault's words have been subjected to different interpretations at different times.

MADNESS

Foucault's first major book (after a somewhat obscure work based on his doctoral thesis) was *Madness and Civilization* (from now abbreviated to *Madness*), first published in French in 1961 followed by an abridged shortened version in English in 1965. The book made its appearance just as questions were being posed about the nature of psychiatry and psychiatric incarceration in Western societies (Goffman's *Asylums* was published in 1961) but it reached Anglophone countries when 'anti-psychiatry' was a growing movement and was rapidly recruited to the anti-psychiatry side. The passage in the book that was seized upon by the anti-psychiatrists was the apparently radical re-interpretation of Pinel's famous act of removing the chains from the mad in Bicetre: removing the chains might have been an act of 'liberation' but only in that it separated the mad from the criminal; more importantly it identified the insane as a new problem and proceeded to subject them to an even more intensive imprisonment. As Sedgewick, an important writer in the field of anti-psychiatry, was later to express it, Foucault's was an 'anti-history of psychiatry'; the new regime was to 'replace the fetters and bars of the old madhouse by the closed, sealed order of an asylum system founded on a gigantic moral imprisonment, that of the medical superintendency of insanity' (1982: 133). In effect, Foucault's account of the history of insanity was seen to undermine the conventional 'progressive' histories of psychiatry, a perspective that was seized upon by those opposed to modern psychiatric incarceration to berate psychiatry's own pretensions to be a progressive and humane discipline. And the example of Pinel provided a model of how to enact another revolution in the care of the mentally ill, only this time patients truly would be liberated from the psychiatric regime that imprisoned them (Ingleby 1980).

The other reading of *Madness* produced by anti-psychiatry was the idea that psychiatric illnesses were 'socially constructed'. There were two facets to this process, both intertwined and never really separated in the sociological literature of the period. On the one hand, mental illness was constructed in the sense of being caused or produced by social activities and conflicts (see, for example, Brown and Harris 1978; Scull 1977); on the other hand, mental illness arose through the definitional processes of psychiatry that labelled some behaviours as normal and others as abnormal (see, for example, Scheff 1966; Szasz 1961). The early formulation of social constructionism that occurred in these debates about psychiatric illness prefigured later applications of this thesis to so-called 'organic' illness but in many ways mental illness was an easier target on which to practise. Whereas physical illnesses could claim a 'real' underpinning in terms of a biological referent, it was clear that psychiatric illness depended very much on the consensual diagnostic practices of psychiatrists that certain illnesses did exist (famously illustrated by the American Psychiatric Association's vote to re-categorise homosexuality as a normal variation rather than a disease).

Not all those in favour of psychiatric reform found *Madness* to their liking. It was either omitted from their analysis of the state of psychiatry or read as a polemical tract by an extremist author (of the Left). Jones, for example, in her original history of the mental health services (published in 1972) makes no mention of Foucault. But by the time of her revised history (1993) published some twenty-one years later, she claimed that *Madness* had exerted a 'massive influence' on sociological thought but only through what she judged as 'an analysis deliberately based on emotive images rather than on logical argument' (1993: 170). Further, she located Foucault on the extreme political left and claimed that he, like Marx, believed that 'capitalism is the sole cause of oppression' (1993: 2). In contrast, Busfield, in her own account of the historical development of madness, found little in *Madness* concerned with asylums and psychiatric practice (others read the book as being precisely about these issues) and thought that Foucault's work could be usefully contrasted with Marxist thought: 'Foucault's lack of direct interest in the extent and nature of the institutions and practices that have arisen to deal with the insane is, therefore, matched by his lack of interest in attempting to link ideas to specific social and economic conditions' (1986: 130). In fact, for Busfield, Foucault's *Madness* was essentially based on the symbolism of insanity producing what she discerned as 'an idealist not a materialistic conception of history' (1986: 130). Yet reading the same text Brown could claim that Foucault showed that 'the creation of the European asylum in the seventeenth and eighteenth centuries [was] a response to the economic dislocation of early industrialism and the political unrest associated with that process' (1985: 13).

In many ways the legacy of *Madness* for sociologists was created in its reading during the anti-psychiatry movement and seems rooted in this period. Reference to the text in most writing in the sociology of health and illness has all but disappeared – though this might also reflect on the relatively low profile of psychiatric disorder in the discipline's literature in the closing years of the century. Other than in explicitly historical accounts of insanity *Madness* is largely ignored. For example, Miles's (1981) book on mental illness in contemporary society makes no reference to Foucault; nor does Prior (1993) in his book on the social organisation of mental illness.

But some of the wider implications of *Madness* that so excited the anti-psychiatrists have been developed by others. Pilgrim and Rogers (1993), for example, in their sociology of mental health and illness, offer a summary of sociological perspectives on psychiatric illness distinguishing between the social causal, the societal reaction and the social constructivist. The last, they charge, has been most strongly influenced by Foucault: 'reality is not self-evident, stable and waiting to be discovered' (1993: 19). And whereas, they suggested, Foucault's early work (in the form of *Madness*) concentrated on the days of 'segregation and "coercive" power', they point to the greater interest of his followers in what they call 'voluntary relationships'.

In my view it is these 'voluntary relationships' that underpin the relevance of *Madness* for the late twentieth (and, no doubt, twenty-first) centuries. In many ways, as I have already argued (Armstrong 1979b), the problem of madness has disappeared just as simply and quickly as it was created by Pinel's liberating gesture. With the post-war policy of de-institutionalisation and legislative changes (including the formal abolition of the term 'insanity') the problem of 'unreason' is also removed from the psychiatric agenda. But this newly vacated psychiatric space did not remain empty for long: a new set of mental health problems have begun to crystallise in the form of the neuroses, the psychological problems of coping with living, the anxieties and depressions of everyday life. This new focus for psychiatric practice – and indeed the wider counselling movement – began to emerge early in the twentieth century and now completely overshadows the old problems of the renamed psychoses. The importance of this shift has been explored in France by Castel (1989) and in Britain notably by Rose (1985, 1990) – though neither of them is identifiable as a sociologist of health and illness. In the main, however, sociologists have largely chosen to concentrate on the social causes of these novel problems and on their distribution in the population/community, rather than explore their 'Foucauldian' origins.

In contrast, medical historians continue to be bemused and exasperated by *Madness*. Arguably, no historical account of psychiatry or of mental illness can ignore a major thesis taken from *Madness*: that not all might be progress in 'improvements' in the management of mental illness. And then there are the historical details of *Madness* that can still provoke historians to arms (Still and Velody 1992). Is *Madness* riven with historical errors? Or is the answer to historians' questions on accuracy contained in the chapters omitted from the English version (Gordon 1992)? Take the noteworthy debate surrounding Foucault's claim that a 'ship of fools' once sailed European waterways. No contemporary evidence, claim some historians, historical reference to such a phenomenon was simply a metaphor for something else, or myths, or distorted readings of texts and so on. But, claim others, this is precisely the point: a 'ship of fools' was a 'reality' but not according to the simplistic notions of historical fact as laid down by professional historians. A problem of language or of translation? (Though even the French historians have to confess the writing in the original is ambiguous.) Whatever its historical 'inaccuracies' this is clearly not a text that historians can ignore.[1]

In summary, the influence of *Madness* is probably greater in history than in sociology. Certainly it has had its adherents who recruited it to the anti-psychiatry movement but with the passing of the asylum and the lower profile given psychoses in recent sociological writing, the effect of *Madness* seems to have waned. However, as in history, some of its broad framework has passed into the sociology of health and illness. Arguably theories of social control and medicalisation have been influenced by the reading that the intervention of the medical profession in areas of human suffering has not always been beneficial; and also its perceived anti-progressivist framework has fed into later 'postmodern' tendencies in the field. Perhaps the ultimate fate of *Madness* is likely to be an ironic one: itself an important reference in a future historiography of unreason.

BIRTH

The Birth of the Clinic (*Birth*) followed *Madness*, published in French in 1963 but having to wait until 1972 for its English translation. Its appearance elicited less excitement than *Madness* and its use by sociologists of health and illness has been much more low key despite the apparent centrality of its subject matter to their concerns. (And if it provokes little interest in health and illness it predictably excites less interest elsewhere. Even Sheridan's [1980] otherwise comprehensive account of the Foucauldian oeuvre is curiously brief in describing the contents of *Birth*.)

Inasmuch as *Birth* claims to be a history of the beginnings of the 'Clinic', that is the cradle of Western hospital or pathological medicine, then it has received a genuflection from those sociologists who wish to argue that such a form of clinical practice is historically and culturally located. Herzlich, for example, in her book on lay representations of health, makes a brief reference to *Birth* as an outstanding example of a text that links together the development of medical science with 'the social conditions from which it emerged' (1973: 6). However the first extended treatment of *Birth* is probably in Illich's *Medical Nemesis* of 1975. In his chapter entitled 'The invention and elimination of disease' Illich states that he draws 'freely from documents gathered in the masterly study [*The Birth of the Clinic*]'. Thereafter, the specific influence of Foucault on Illich's polemic is more difficult to determine; perhaps his reference to the contemporary documentation that Foucault had gathered together in *Birth* reflects an indebtedness to sources rather than the interpretation of that material.

During the 1980s and 1990s *Birth* has been used in two ways within the sociology of health and illness. First, it seems to have a useful and relatively uncontroversial role as an easy reference to quote to cover the sweep of the early history of Western or hospital medicine (and performs a similar function for historians who have been less critical of its historical 'accuracy' than they were of *Madness*). Mention Western medicine, bio-medicine, the clinic, pathological medicine, or some other synonym and a citation of *Birth* performs a useful support function (the first time I referenced *Birth* in my own work was in this abbreviated way, see Armstrong 1979a). Such a reference is a safe one to make: it indicates that Western medicine is both historically and culturally located (not much to disagree about there), but beyond that requires no commitment or involvement in any other aspect of Foucauldian disputation.

Second, and less ritualistic, is the use of the 'medical gaze' that frequently emerges as a central theme of Foucault's text. The ground has been well covered: the original French '*le regard*' was translated as 'perception' for the sub-title and as 'the gaze' in the main body of the text. Neither translation on its own fully captures the subtlety of '*le regard*', at once a perception but also an active mode of seeing. The gaze has been identified by a number of different writers as representing the process through which specific social objects, namely disease categories, come into existence and how more recent shifts can be seen as changes in the gaze (Armstrong 1983; Nettleton 1992; Thornquist 1995). A particular example of the genre is Atkinson's (1981) study of medical student socialisation in which he describes the processes through which the artistry of the gaze is communicated to neophytes. One result of these analyses has been 'social construction-ism' or 'constructivism'. Here, even more than in *Madness*, it can be argued that Foucault's work has been a major influence on the constructionist heresy in sociology of health and illness (whilst recognising that social constructionism has other roots and appears independently of Foucault in cognate disciplines such as in the sociology of science and in psychology). Indeed it is not uncommon to write about the social construction of the body with no reference to Foucault (Nicholson and McLaughlin 1987) or only a passing one (Freund and McGuire 1995).

But, as is well recognised, social constructionism is a broad church and even those drawing inspiration from Foucault's original arrive at different conclusions. For example, Prior observes in his study of death in Belfast that it was Foucault who made the fundamental point that the body was historically and culturally located; this meant that 'The body, therefore, does not and cannot yield its essential features to naked observation unmediated by forms of knowledge' (1989: 13). Yet he implies that there are 'essential features' of the body, independent of the 'gaze'. Others, such as myself and Nettleton (1992), have been more relativistic on this point: if the body can only be known through a descriptive language (the 'gaze' for the last two centuries) then it is futile to speculate on 'essential features' that could never be described.

While *Birth* provided an important conceptual framework for some writers in terms of a 'way of seeing' for understanding how Western medicine was able to identify diseases deep in the body, it has probably proved most fruitful when this insight has been combined with themes of surveillance and power that are described in Foucault's later work. However, the rest of *Birth*, to my mind, has been little exploited. It is dense and, as it is focused on a few decades two centuries ago, it can appear more suited to the interests of historians. But it displays a glittering prose style that begs for recitation. I am afraid that a lecture or seminar that includes *Birth* can rapidly degenerate into a sermon as the master's words are read out loud. And besides the poetry I also find the book full of nuggets that can be easily mined. For example, I have found an analytic tool in the use of spaces for exploring the distributions of illness in geriatric medicine (Armstrong 1981a), or in the identification of spaces – conceptual, social, geographic, temporal – in modern British general practice (Armstrong 1993, 1985). Indeed, Foucault's opening differentiation of primary, secondary and tertiary spatialisation of illness (a sort of cognitive, corporal and geographic map) provides an excellent device for explaining more recent changes in the nature of illness (Armstrong 1993, 1995).

I have also found value in reading about the meaning of death. 'Man does not die because he falls ill; he falls ill because he might die' allows death itself to be seen as a social construction interwoven with particular models of illness. Thus, as I read it, Foucault suggested that death was a natural phenomenon in the eighteenth century (only the coroner's court determining 'unnatural' causes such as murder or misfortune) but became a pathological event in the nineteenth (and twentieth) century with the concomitant rise of hospital medicine and the post-mortem to establish the pathological cause of death. (I still tease medical students with the question: is death normal or abnormal?) This analysis gave me the framework to explore the construction of infant deaths during the final decades of the nineteenth and twentieth centuries (Armstrong 1986). It also, together with ideas from a later text, allowed me to explore a mid-twentieth-century change in the nature of death (Armstrong 1987).

But perhaps the most profound lesson I take from *Birth* is the subtext on the emergence of the individual. The patient appears at various points as a repository for this new model of a pathology-based disease. The patient in this sense is no more than a container for the lesion; but it seems that this undistinguished container is one form in which individual identity begins to make its appearance on the Western stage. The very idea of separate identity, albeit in prototype and anatomical form, begins to emerge for me from these pages: sometimes there seems explicit reference, as in Foucault's discussion of the relationship between the individual and death, but it is in the brief concluding chapter that he suggests out loud, so to speak, that the deployment of the clinical gaze forms an integral part of our individual experience and identity. This belief that medicine has an important role in fabricating individual experience and identity has been an important one for me and has underpinned many of my writings. For example, it was hardly a major step to move from my reading of Foucault on this point to an exploration of the further development of the individual through the advice on interrogating/interviewing patients contained in clinical manuals published during the twentieth century (Armstrong 1984).

DISCIPLINE

While I found that *Birth* had a tendency to overwhelm by its detail, the strength of *Discipline and Punish* (*Discipline*) was the simplicity and clarity of its main thesis. Published in French in 1975 and in English in 1977 it seemed instantly accessible; for me, working on a thesis on medical knowledge and the medical division of labour (1981b), later published as *Political Anatomy of the Body* (1983), it was a godsend. I read it as contextualising his previous books: here he described a shift from sovereign to disciplinary power that seemed to fit with key historical shifts identified in his earlier works. And in the idea of surveillance as the underlying mechanism of disciplinary power, Foucault seemed to strike a chord for many other readers.

Three types of research have subsequently been published in the sociology of health and illness that have utilised notions of surveillance and power. First, there are those 'historical' studies that have in common the use of the idea of historical shifts in surveillance/power, as in *Discipline*, as the main explanation for the emergence of new medical phenomena. Thus, Arney (1982) and Arney and Bergen (1984) found it of value in understanding the post-war explosion in obstetric technology and in recent trends in clinical practice respectively; Nettleton used it as the basis for explaining the emergence of teeth and the mouth over the last century (1992); and I have used it a number of times as the basic map that guides my own explorations of some of these issues. (Though when Osborne [1994] revisited some of the topics that I had found of interest with his own reading of Foucault he judged my work to be too pessimistic and overly determined.)

The second group of studies, increasing in number, are qualitative investigations into aspects of interaction in medical settings. While these have often relied on apparently inductive approaches, they have begun to see surveillance – and its effects – as a recurrent theme. For example, Silverman (1987) used ideas of surveillance to understand the broader context in which clinics function; Daly (1989) found the idea of surveillance, and resistance to surveillance, significant in her study of echocardiography; similarly Bloor and McIntosh (1990) found the tension between surveillance and concealment a valuable frame-work for explaining interactions in the community between professionals and their clients. Less surprisingly perhaps, the Foucauldian notion of surveillance also has more immediate resonances in those parts of medicine that are, by their own admission, concerned with surveillance; for example, in dental check-ups (Nettleton 1988), in cervical screening (McKie 1995) and in health promotion (Bunton 1992; Petersen 1996).

The third type of output to include the theme of surveillance/power is that which attempts to state or develop a more theoretical argument for the sociology of health and illness than the more empirically based studies described above. These run from the undergraduate textbooks that try and locate the Foucauldian perspective (often under the constructionist label) as one of several theoretical perspectives in the sociology of health and illness (for example, Morgan *et al.* 1985). Others have tried more ambitiously to develop and extend Foucault; however, these have all read Foucault in different ways and therefore achieve different outcomes. Gerhardt (1989), in an ambitious intellectual history of medical sociology, places Foucault, along with the Marxists, in a 'conflict-theory paradigm'. In contrast, Fox (1993a) locates Foucault as a postmodern author but still subsumes him to other better recognised figures from that arena. But perhaps the best-known exposition of the Foucault influence on the sociology of health and illness is the work of Turner.

Besides a number of papers (and books on other subjects) Turner has engaged with Foucault in three main texts, namely *The Body and Society* (1984), *Medical Power and Social Knowledge* (1987) and *Regulating Bodies* (1992). Turner's main argument is that the body has been essentially 'absent' from social theory and his aim is to make it a central feature. In part this has involved the 'application of the philosophy of Michel Foucault' to the problem of the body, but he has also brought to bear the work of other theorists. As Turner himself explained, this has meant that he has 'often been criticised for eclecticism, and for a lack of theoretical integration' (1992: 4) – though he felt that this view was partly the product of the diversity of projects that he had pursued. The result of this eclecticism in *The Body and Society*, by Turner's own admission, was a predominantly Marxist framework – and Foucault was 'integrated' into this. For example, Turner felt that 'Foucault's project can be seen to bear a relationship to a view of historical materialism presented by Engels' (1984: 35). This Marxist framework continued into the 1987 text: for example, Turner placed great emphasis on the importance of Foucault's radical notion of power but proceeded to suggest that 'The clinical gaze enabled medical men to assume considerable social power in defining reality and hence in identifying deviance and social disorder' (1987: 11).

By the time of his 1992 text, again apparently strongly influenced by Foucault, he acknowledged that 'a Marxist problematic was relatively dominant in *The Body and Society* and that a decade later these arguments look somewhat dated' (1992: 6). Indeed, in retrospect, he felt that *The Body and Society* had 'brought to a conclusion a period in my own intellectual development, which had been heavily influenced by the sociologies of Karl Marx and Max Weber' (1992: 5). The stage was thus set for a re-interpretation of Foucault: 'Now that the full scope and scale of his work [following his death] can be more adequately appreciated and understood, my original use of his approach appears in retrospect to be inadequate' (1992: 7). However, the new look was not Marx but Weber. Foucauldian ideas on power and surveillance were 'to my mind parallel to Weberian categories of rationalisation and disenchantment' (1992: 10), claimed Turner. Indeed, he now pointed out that in *The Body and Society* he had made similar claims, arguing that his own previous work denied the originality of Foucault's thesis by bringing out certain continuities between Weber's notion of 'rationalisation' and Foucault's discussion of 'disciplines' (1984: 2).

Clearly Turner has himself made a number of readings of Foucault, particularly in terms of the theoretical tradition in which he locates him. Yet there are some common features of these readings that are at odds with the work of others, in particular my own work. To my mind the gaze of the clinic and the surveillance machinery of the Panopticon fabricated bodies and the diseases that were contained within them. But Turner would see limits to this argument. Again his eclecticism allows him to bring in sociobiology as part of his explanatory framework (surely itself demanding explanation?): 'While human society has change [sic] fundamentally over the last 2000 years, sociobiology would suggest that the human body has remained, in all important respects, physiologically static' (1984: 35). His biological reductionism comes through more fully when he tackles directly the social construction of disease: 'It appears bizarre to argue that there are no organic foundations to human activity' (1992: 16); he goes on: 'For example, it is unlikely that a human being will ever outrun a horse over a mile in fair conditions; if the front legs of the horse are not tied together!' (1992: 16). These statements might seem to fit uneasily with Turner's oft-repeated assertion that 'the body is socially constructed', but for Turner 'some things ("hysteria") may be more socially constructed than others ("gout")' (1992: 26). Given the stated importance of Foucault's writings for Turner it might be assumed that claims such as the above (that seem to privilege knowledge provided by the biological sciences) are somehow rooted in a biological reductionist reading of Foucault, though they might equally represent yet another facet of his eclecticism.

The shifting nature of Turner's position as well as his view of Foucault as a neo-Marxist or a neo-Weberian illustrates the different readings of Foucault that are possible. Certainly many writers have tried to fuse him to a Marxist position or locate him within a 'great tradition' of sociological theorists (my [1985] contribution to this search for origins managed to discover great affinities to Durkheim!); others have taken his texts as more of a radical break with the past.

HISTORY

The *History of Sexuality, Volume 1* (*History*) was published in 1976 and translated into English in 1978. Like *Madness*, its instant appeal seemed to lie in its overturning of conventional assumptions. The nineteenth century had not been a period of repression but one of incitement to talk about and discuss sexuality. In this sense, like disease in *Birth*, sexuality was a product of discourse or, more correctly, discursive practices. This thesis has proved a powerful one, especially in an era of AIDS, but its impact on the sociology of health and illness has been relatively slight. Turner tried to link the sociology of the body with the sociology of sex and claimed that the failure to engage with the latter was one good reason for 'taking Foucault seriously' (1984: 9). Yet his appeal has not been taken up with enthusiasm, perhaps because sociologists of health and illness *per se* have been less concerned with researching sexuality.

Nevertheless, I think that there are other themes to be quarried from this slim book, in particular a more extensive description of what is meant by power within a disciplinary regime. It still might be less than totally transparent but to my mind the dozen pages following Foucault's claim that 'we have yet to cut off the head of the king' offer a provocative and novel way of looking at power. This has underpinned some of my own work: for example, the shift in regimes of public health that I identified seems to tie in well with underlying mechanisms of power, from the role of sovereignty in maintaining the traditional *cordon sanitaire* to the disciplinary power implied by the new public health and its message of individualised risk and ecological purity. Even so this reading is by no means common and many writers, such as Turner, take

Foucault to be describing new mechanisms for operating more traditional power as possessed by individuals or interests. For example, Anderson *et al.* see the power to normalise conferring new powers on those who hold that power: 'Foucault would have us see power diffused throughout society, and the oppressors not as a faceless "ruling class", but psychiatrists, physicians, managers and the like' (1989: 274).

While the overt linking of power/resistance with sexuality might have seemed more relevant for the literature on the latter topic, there is another theme that had been read in Foucault's earlier work but was now placed in a seemingly wider theoretical perspective, and this was subjectivity. The fabrication of bodies in *Birth* and *Discipline* could so easily be linked to the wider problems of identity; but here in *History* the linkage seemed more explicit. Studies of power/resistance in clinical settings might sometimes reference 'earlier' Foucault but seem to depend on the 'clarifications' offered in *History*. A good example is the work of Lupton, particularly in her analysis of public health (1995), also Fox (1993b) on the emergence of subjectivity, and May (1992) on the problem of subjectivity in nursing, as well as many of the studies mentioned above.

On a more personal note, I was also impressed by the way in which Foucault handled the 'undercurrent' of sexual discourse that was incited by the Victorians yet has continued to our own day, in particular his claim that 'silence' was not the opposite of discourse but another facet of it. It made me recall Ariès's claim that discourse on death had been silenced for a hundred years between the mid-nineteenth and mid-twentieth centuries. Could this be given the Foucault treatment too? Rather than repression about death, an incitement to discourse? And rather than late twentieth-century liberation the imposition of a new regime of truth? Yes, the new and massive discourse on death within medicine fitted almost exactly into the period of so-called silence. And the new requirement from the 1960s that the dying should mourn their own deaths fitted the point of so-called liberation (Armstrong 1987).

CONCLUSION

This has been a personal reading at many levels. It is a personal reading, or perhaps re-reading, of some of my own work; indulgent perhaps, but only to pay homage. Foucault's texts have been a constant source of inspiration and, as I have tried to make clear, a cornucopia of ideas and frameworks that I have unashamedly stolen: it is reassuring to think that he might not have existed and therefore cannot take umbrage at these thefts acknowledged only casually by the conventional superscript and bibliographic reference.

The essay is also a personal reading of the work of others. And as in the debate over the ship of fools, others have read sentences and concepts differently. Sometimes I have liked their reading, other times I think they have missed the pearls. Nevertheless Foucault does seem to have been an important influence, perhaps more cited over the last decade than any other theoretical source.

Finally, this essay is a personal reading of Foucault. Like everyone else, I have been reading Foucault and reading readers of Foucault through a prism in which text and reader are simultaneously refracted and reflected. The exact source of the light is therefore unclear, but this is not a problem that should seriously concern us.

NOTE

1 See David McCallum's chapter (chapter 3) for further discussion of 'Foucault the historian', with particular reference to *Madness*.

REFERENCES

Anderson, J.M., Elfert, H. and Lai, M. (1989) 'Ideology in the clinical context: chronic illness, ethnicity and the discourse on normalisation', *Sociology of Health & Illness*, 11: 253–78.

Armstrong, D. (1979a) 'The emancipation of biographical medicine', *Social Science and Medicine*, 13: 1–8.

Armstrong, D. (1979b) 'Madness and coping', *Sociology of Health & Illness*, 2: 293–316.

Armstrong, D. (1981a) 'Pathological life and death', *Social Science and Medicine*, 15: 253–7.

Armstrong, D. (1981b) 'Developments in medical thought and practice in the twentieth century', Unpublished PhD thesis, London University.

Armstrong, D. (1983) *Political Anatomy of the Body: Medical Knowledge in Britain in the Twentieth Century*, Cambridge: Cambridge University Press.

Armstrong, D. (1984) 'The patient's view', *Social Science and Medicine*, 18: 737–44.

Armstrong, D. (1985) 'Space and time in British general practice', *Social Science and Medicine*, 20: 659–66.

Armstrong, D. (1986) 'The invention of infant mortality', *Sociology of Health & Illness*, 8: 211–32.

Armstrong, D. (1987) 'Silence and truth in death and dying', *Social Science and Medicine*, 24: 651–7.

Armstrong, D. (1993) 'Public health spaces and the fabrication of identity', *Sociology*, 27: 393–410.

Armstrong, D. (1995) 'The rise of surveillance medicine', *Sociology of Health & Illness*, 17: 393–404.

Arney, W.R. (1982) *Power and the Profession of Obstetrics*, Chicago: University of Chicago Press.

Arney, W.R. and Bergen, B.J. (1984) *Medicine and the Management of Living*, Chicago: University of Chicago Press.

Atkinson, P. (1981) *The Clinical Experience: The Construction and Reconstruction of Medical Student Reality*, Farnborough: Gower.

Bloor, M. and McIntosh, J. (1990) 'Surveillance and concealment: a comparison of techniques of client resistance in therapeutic communities and health visiting', in S. Cunningham-Burley and N. McKeganey (eds) *Readings in Medical Sociology*, London: Tavistock.

Brown, G.W. and Harris, T. (1978) *Social Origins of Depression*, London: Tavistock.

Brown, P. (1985) *The Transfer of Care: Psychiatric De-institutionalisation and its Aftermath*, London: Routledge.

Bunton, R. (1992) 'More than a woolly jumper: health promotion as social regulation', *Critical Public Health*, 3, 2: 4–11.

Busfield, J. (1986) *Managing Madness: Changing Ideas and Practice*, London: Hutchinson.

Castel, R. (1989) *The Psychiatric Order*, Cambridge: Polity Press.

Daly, J. (1989) 'Innocent murmurs: echocardiography and the diagnosis of cardiac normality', *Sociology of Health & Illness*, 11: 99–116.

Foucault, M. (1965) *Madness and Civilization*, New York: Random House.

Foucault, M. (1973) *The Birth of the Clinic: An Archaeology of Medical Perception*, London: Tavistock.

Foucault, M. (1977) *Discipline and Punish: The Birth of the Prison*, London: Allen Lane.

Foucault, M. (1979) *The History of Sexuality, Volume 1: An Introduction*, London: Allen Lane.

Fox, N.J. (1993a) *Post-modernism, Sociology and Health*, Buckingham: Open University Press.

Fox, N.J. (1993b) 'Discourse, organisation and the surgical ward round', *Sociology of Health & Illness*, 15: 16–42.

Freund, P.S. and McGuire, M.B. (1995) *Health, Illness and the Social Body*, Englewood Cliffs, NJ: Prentice Hall.

Gerhardt, U. (1989) *Ideas about Illness*, London: Macmillan.

Goffman, E. (1961) *Asylums*, London: Allen Lane.

Gordon, C. (1992) '*Histoire de la folie*: an unknown book by Michel Foucault', in A. Still and I. Velody (eds) *Rewriting the History of Madness*, London: Routledge.

Herzlich, C. (1973) *Health and Illness: A Social Psychological Analysis*, London: Academic Press.

Illich, I. (1975) *Medical Nemesis*, London: Calder and Boyars.

Ingleby, D. (1980) *Critical Psychiatry: The Politics of Mental Health*, New York: Pantheon.

Jones, K. (1972) *A History of the Mental Health Services*, London: Routledge.

Jones, K. (1993) *Asylums and After: A Revised History of the Mental Health Services: From the Early Eighteenth Century to the 1990s*, London: Athlone.

Lupton, D. (1995) *The Imperative of Health: Public Health and the Regulated Body*, London: Sage.

May, C. (1992) 'Nursing work, nurses' knowledge, and the subjectification of the patient', *Sociology of Health & Illness*, 14: 472–87.

McKie, L. (1995) 'The art of surveillance or reasonable prevention? The case of cervical screening', *Sociology of Health & Illness*, 17: 441–57.

Miles, A. (1981) *The Mentally Ill in Contemporary Society*, Oxford: Martin Robertson.

Morgan, M., Calnan, M. and Manning, N. (1985) *Sociological Approaches to Health and Medicine*, London: Croom Helm.

Nettleton, S. (1988) 'Protecting a vulnerable margin: towards an analysis of how the mouth came to be separated from the body', *Sociology of Health & Illness*, 10: 156–69.

Nettleton, S. (1992) *Power, Pain and Dentistry*, Buckingham: Open University Press.

Nicholson, M. and McLaughlin, C. (1987) 'Social constructionism and medical sociology: a reply to M.R. Bury', *Sociology of Health & Illness*, 9: 107–26.

Osborne, T. (1994) 'Power and persons: on ethical stylisation and person-centred medicine', *Sociology of Health & Illness*, 16: 515–35.

Petersen, A.R. (1996) 'Risk and the regulated self: the discourse of health promotion as politics of uncertainty', *Australian & New Zealand Journal of Sociology*, 32, 1: 44–57.

Pilgrim, D. and Rogers, A. (1993) *A Sociology of Mental Health and Illness*, Buckingham: Open University Press.

Prior, L. (1989) *The Social Organisation of Death: Medical Discourse and Social Practices in Belfast*, London: Macmillan.

Prior, L. (1993) *The Social Organisation of Mental Illness*, London: Sage.

Rose, N. (1985) *The Psychological Complex*, London: Routledge and Kegan Paul.

Rose, N. (1990) *Governing the Soul: The Shaping of the Private Self*, London: Routledge.

Scheff, T. (1966) *Being Mentally Ill: A Sociological Theory*, Chicago: Aldine.

Scull, A.T. (1977) *Decarceration*, Englewood Cliffs, NJ: Prentice Hall.

Sedgewick, P. (1982) *Psychopolitics*, London: Pluto Press.

Sheridan, A. (1980) *Michel Foucault: The Will to Truth*, London: Tavistock.

Silverman, D. (1987) *Communication and Medical Practice*, London: Sage.

Still, A. and Velody, I. (1992) *Rewriting the History of Madness*, London: Routledge.

Szasz, T. (1961) *The Myth of Mental Illness: Foundations of a Theory of Personal Conduct*, New York: Hoeber-Harper.

Thornquist, E. (1995) 'Musculoskeletal suffering: a diagnosis and a variant view', *Sociology of Health & Illness*, 17: 166–92.

Turner, B.S. (1984) *The Body and Society: Explorations in Social Theory*, Oxford: Blackwell.

Turner, B.S. (1987) *Medical Power and Social Knowledge*, London: Sage.

Turner, B.S. (1992) *Regulating Bodies: Essays in Medical Sociology*, London: Routledge.

Chapter 2

Is there life after Foucault?

Texts, frames and *differends*

Nick J. Fox

INTRODUCTION: THE FAR SIDE OF FOUCAULT

When post-structuralism is applied to social theory, its epistemology contributes some new perspectives on agency and structure, change and continuity (Game 1991; Fox 1993). In particular, it contributes an understanding of the relationship between 'power' and 'knowledge', of the discursive construction of the self as opposed to a more essential conception, and a recognition of difference and diversity both as (dis)organising principles and as the basis for ethics and politics (Haber 1994). It would be fair to say that the impact of post-structuralism and postmodern philosophy within social theory has been dominated over the past decade by the position developed by Michel Foucault (Valverde 1991: 184; Lupton 1994: 5), a claim borne out by the contributions to this volume. However, closer examination of this 'sociological Foucault' which emerges in Foucauldian studies suggests that – while the epistemology has been embraced and used productively – the full complexities of the ontological implications of the de-centring of self and the 'deep structure' conception of the rules of discursive formation deserve closer attention. Part of this chapter will be devoted to such explorations.

My argument will be that Foucault's ontology is sometimes ambiguous and contradictory. While such ambiguity is not necessarily a fatal flaw (perhaps indeed it is an antidote to modernist meta-narrative), I will suggest that, in terms of clarity, engagement with sociological theory and application to field settings, there is some virtue to be found in exploring other positions deriving from post-structuralism and postmodern theory, to see if there is 'life after Foucault'. I am going to develop one such perspective, in terms of principles concerning *texts* and *framing* which draw on postmodern writers including Roland Barthes, Jacques Derrida and Jean-François Lyotard. As will be seen, this approach de-emphasises Foucault's concern with the historical genealogy of knowledge and subjectivity, instead developing perspectives on intertextuality which may be used to study many areas within the purview of social theory. Because my background is in the study of health and illness, my critique of Foucauldian ontology and the development of this other perspective engage with examples taken primarily from that field; however, the application may be made in other areas within social theory.

TEXTS AND FRAMES

Intertextuality is the process whereby one text plays upon other texts, in the endless referentiality of texts and other elements of cultural production (Barthes 1977). It is a feature of all texts – given that a text is defined as a meaningful symbolic system. Three statements serve to generate the basics of what I shall call the 'texts and framing' (henceforth TF) position.

1   In the study of the social, the primary unit of analysis is the *text*, which may be writing, bodily or social practice, or subjective sense-of-self, to which meaning may be ascribed. Texts are the product of human activity; as such they are created within the flow of history, yet they are fragmentary, they are continually re-read and have no single or final meaning.
2   Texts engage with each other productively, and in this *intertextuality*, meaning comes into being, is sustained, distorted, obscured or re-introduced. The capacity to engage meaningfully with the social world – that is, to understand and to contribute to that world – is intertextual, a function of a subjectivity which is itself textual and not prior to textuality.
3   The meaning of a text resides in its *frame*, that is, in that which distinguishes and separates it from what it is not. Power is a phenomenon of the frame: to write the limits of a text is a political act. But the framing is always provisional, subject to challenge and re-negotiation, and is always in the process of being achieved.

In intertextual approaches, the emphasis is upon the reader rather than the writer: a displacement of great significance for understanding power, knowledge and resistance. While texts are written by humans, their writers' *authorship* is provisional: authority is observable only at its site of action; that is, at the site of *reading*. Bodies of 'knowledge' are thus a feature of reception rather than authorship, while resistance becomes possible in the re-reading (and hence rewriting) of texts as readers substantiate or discredit the discourses with which they engage. While intertextuality is implicit in Foucault, its working through becomes possible only when reception of texts becomes seen as an active process rather than a passive 'inscription'. In place of the determinism of a focus which privileges discourse and the authority which it supplies, there is an opening up of as many possibilities for human becoming as there are intertexts (a number which, in theory, is infinite).

One feature of intertextuality is that it will contribute endlessly not only to knowledge or 'ideology', but also to that text which we call 'subjectivity' or sense-of-self. Using the notion of *framing* to explore this further, subjectivity comes to be seen as something dynamic, always in flux as intertextual readings contribute to a continuous process of *becoming-other*. Framing is the making sense of otherwise meaningless patternings of signs – it is the *gestalt* which imposes meaning and privileges certain interpretations over others. Deleuze and Guattari (1984, 1988) spoke of a 'nomadic subjectivity' potentially free to wander through textuality, although always drawn to one *plateau* (framing) or another. Framing as such is an active process – a making-sense activity which like a neural net (a computer simulation of human information-processing) patterns data in ways which provide the potential for the ascription of meaning. In turn, this process of making sense out of non-sense is what makes it possible for us to engage with the world reflexively (rather than simply responding to it in a Skinnerian sense).

Subjectivity is thus tied up with this reading of texts, and the dynamism of subjectivity is a feature of intertextuality, the play of text on text, sign upon sign. In the same way that a neural net computer program can 'learn' from the information which is introduced to it – so that it responds in predictable ways to new information and yet is able to modify its behaviour dependent on that information – the framing of texts creates a continuity to experience, although the flow of textuality makes such framings provisional and capable of re-framing. Re-framing is thus both a 'reading' and a 'writing', and what is read and written is, in part, the self. The self is not prior: in this sense, texts read the self rather than being read by it.

This is not to imply that intertextual subjectivity is free to become whatever it may. In practice, framings are constrained in all sorts of ways. For Lyotard (1988), oppositional politics can be understood as a play of texts: 'phrases in dispute' or *differends*, all seeking to gain authority over the others. When one phrase gains ascendancy, it is by the (rhetorical) denial of the intertextuality which might enable opposing discourses to 'prove' their own positions. As such, the *differend* is a marker of the violence which is done in the name of discourse, the victimisation of the position in submission (Lyotard 1988: 9). The significance of such *differends* will be seen in the example offered later in this chapter. A *differend* can be sustained only by the consistent distancing of proponent and subject, by the refusal to admit that a subject might be able to speak. A *differend*, in other words, is a constraint upon intertextuality. While such a constraint may be imposed from outside of the discourse itself – by the threat of sanctions or the use of other resources in the psychological or social world of the subject – the aim of discursive practices, understood in this way, is to sustain this distantiation between the proponent of discourse and its subject-matter. Foucault's *gaze* of power is an example of such distantiation between the subject of the gaze and the object – the body (Game 1991: 42).

The creation of the differend, and thus of what Foucault calls discourse, is an act of framing: discourse acts at its margin or limit, where it creates distance between author and object, self and other, what is and what is not. In *The Truth in Painting*, Derrida (1987) suggests that authorial intent (albeit subject to continual re-reading) engages with its reader/observer not through the content of a text, but by its *frame*. Where the limits of a text are positioned, how it is framed in relationship to that which is beyond it, what is thus excluded, is as important as what is included in a text or textual practice.

I have drawn upon post-structuralists other than Foucault in this exegesis of the TF position, primarily Barthes, Derrida, Deleuze and Guattari and Lyotard. Up to a point, I could have recruited Foucault in this exploration, in particular around his rejection of the notion of the author (Foucault 1977a) and of the patterning of discourse and its relation to nomadic subjectivity (1977c). But I have tried to set out a position which – ontologically – depends on nothing other than the capacity of the human brain to process information according to *gestalts* which I suggest can be understood as 'framings'. In this sense, there are substantial differences in terms of ontology between the TF position and Foucault's more complex ontology as demonstrated in his writings and in those of his 'followers' within social theory. To illustrate these differences, and – I hope – make the case for this alternative perspective, I need to engage with Foucauldian ontology.

The next three sections critically address the characteristics of this ontology in terms of three areas: discourse, the body and the self. Subsequently, I will return to the TF, to look more closely at its ontologies of these areas, with recourse to an example of its application in the social theory of health and illness.

FOUCAULT'S ONTOLOGY OF DISCOURSE

Foucault's central concern is with power (Foucault 1981: 115), and he is critical of theories which consider power as 'sovereign': a unitary and centralised construct (Wickham 1986: 169) and hence primarily repressive in character. A principal technology of power, argues Foucault (1976, 1979, 1980a), is the *gaze*, which is concerned with the gathering of information, to inform and create a discourse on its subject-matter. Discourses create *effects of truth* which are of themselves neither true nor false (Foucault 1980b: 116–19). Because of this association of a productive power with the fabrication of effects of truth, Foucault speaks of *power/knowledge* – a phenomenon which cannot be reduced simply to either component. It has been argued that Foucault's ontology breaks both with structuralism and with humanism (Dreyfus and Rabinow 1982; Smart 1985: 16). It breaks (but incompletely, I will argue) with structuralism in that it denies that power is something which is merely coercive in a traditional Marxist or Weberian perspective (Pizzorno 1992). It marks a break with humanism inasmuch as it de-centres the individual as the prior agent in creating the social world, rejecting subjectivity as something essential, prior to discourse, which power acts against. Power is a productive process, creating human subjects and their capacity to act (Butler 1990: 139).

The centrality of the concept of discourse in Foucault's work, and its association with knowledge and power, suggest a continuity between his project, the sociology of knowledge and the method in social psychology known as discourse analysis. However, the term 'discourse' is used in a very specific way by Foucault. Foucault sought to develop a basis for understanding what makes knowledge possible, to attempt an 'archaeology' of knowledge, underpinned by 'rules' which operate independently of subjectivity (Foucault 1974: 15–16). Three aspects of Foucault's ontology of discourse can be identified.

First, while subjects may be capable of interpreting the surface meanings of discursive practices, and thus developing a contingent 'knowledge', the 'deeper' knowledge is not directly accessible, mainly because it is not knowledge at all in the everyday sense of the word. The system of rules which govern the production, operation and regulation of discursive statements (the surface level) mediates *power* or more precisely a 'will to power': not the will of one particular person or group but a generalised will to create the possibilities to be able to 'speak the truth' (Hacking 1986: 34–5). The will to power is productive, of 'new ways of saying plausible things about other human beings and ourselves'. Subjectivity (that is, the ability to know oneself) is itself achieved through discourse (as the child of a deeper 'power/knowledge'), clarifying why a prior, privileged or essential subject must be unacceptable within a Foucauldian framework (Nettleton 1992: 132).

Second, Foucault recognises discursive practices as human activity, 'embodied in technical processes, in institutions, in patterns for general behaviour, in forms for transmission and diffusion, and in pedagogical forms which, at once, impose and maintain them' (Foucault 1977b: 200). However, not all human activity or other events are discursive. Most 'real' historical events or pieces of human behaviour are what Foucault calls 'non-discursive practices', and the relationship between discourse and the non-discursive is not simply a mirroring, in which discourse is the surface manifestation of 'reality' (Brown and Cousins 1986: 36). Rather, discourse is the surface manifestation of the underlying will to power (which Foucault calls 'power/knowledge' in his later work) which cannot be reduced to human intentionality (Brown and Cousins 1986: 37–8). Indeed, power/knowledge is that which links discourse to the non-discursive, that creates the connections which makes it possible to speak about some aspect of the world in a particular regime of truth. That which is non-discursive plays no part in such regimes, and whether or not it becomes discursive cannot be determined from essential features of the event itself.

Third, if power/knowledge is unknowable in a traditional sense, then it follows that no one or no group such as the sovereign, the bourgeoisie or the state can (intentionally) be its author or possess it absolutely (Foucault 1980c: 98). Neither is discourse something which coincides necessarily with single works or groups of works or even specific disciplines. Discourse in this sense has a life of its own independent of human agency (Foucault 1977b: 200–1), and cannot be reduced to particular texts or practices. It is also clear that, given the unknowability of power/knowledge, discerning its 'hidden meaning' could not be the objective of analysis, Foucauldian or otherwise.

This ontology of discourse is quite different from humanist sociological notions of the structuring of agency (Smart 1985: 71; Hacking 1986: 35). To summarise, discourse cannot be reduced to texts or other 'authored' practices, does not directly mirror the 'reality' of historical events (the non-discursive), and is the surface manifestation of a deeper power/knowledge, which is anonymous, is disseminated and cannot be known in a traditional sense. Nor is discourse simply a new way of thinking about social structure, which in traditional social theory – however deterministic – can always be 'explained' (as roles, the economic base or whatever): Foucault's conception of discourse is radically divorced, both from 'reality' and from traditional notions of human subjectivity. It follows that strategies appropriate to a humanistic framework, for instance recourse to authorial intention, historical events or contexts, cannot be adopted when utilising this model.

The unfamiliarity of such a notion of an ahistorical, non-authored discourse governed by a free-floating, anonymous, disseminated power/ knowledge requires most cautious methodological rigour when applied within social analysis. It is fairly clear that Foucault was aware of the potential for an essentialism of power (Freundlieb 1994: 158–62), and he argues that power is 'an open more-or-less co-ordinated (in the event, no doubt, ill-co-ordinated) cluster of relations' (Foucault 1980d: 199). At the level of the rules governing discourse, it is a principle of 'dispersion' (or what might be called difference) rather than unity which holds sway (Freundlieb 1994: 162). However, Wickham discerns a tendency to essentialise power/knowledge as unitary and pre-existing in Foucault's own commentary on the way in which power used the law to achieve legitimacy (1986: 152–7). It is unsurprising that from time to time a notion of power as something which is itself an agent and can 'use' discourse emerges in Foucauldian studies. So, for example, Armstrong writes that

> Panoptic power had fabricated bodies by making them the objects of an observing eye. The new regime exercised surveillance over the whole population and, because it observed the mind of everyone, was in a better position to make the individual a point of articulation for power: both an effect of power and a point from which power was exercised.
>
> (Armstrong 1983: 70)

At the extreme, power/knowledge becomes synonymous with 'the state' or 'society' or some particular grouping, reflecting a functionalism which can sometimes be discerned in *Discipline and Punish* (Donnelly 1986: 29; Hoy 1986: 7–8). The relations of power are brought into such close allegiance with the grouping in whose interest power works that we are back with sovereign (essential) power (Wickham 1986: 171–2).

While this tendency to essentialise power/knowledge as unitary, sovereign and (because it is absurd to imagine power as in and of itself capable of agency) potentially the possession of a person or persons thus introduces human agency through the back door, a second tendency re-introduces humanism elsewhere: through the authorial voice of the texts which contribute to discourse. Foucault's later writing is less concerned with the archaeology of the 'rules' of discursive formation than with the *genealogy* of power/knowledge: the changing relationship of discourse to the non-discursive over time (Smart 1985: 42), in other words to the objects of history – in particular, bodies, selves and subjectivity in general.

Foucault's genealogies draw more heavily on the surface manifestations of discursive practices, the human productions of texts or non-textual practices, and there is thus the potential for any text or practice to be labelled 'discursive', eliding the distinction between written texts and 'discourse', between which Foucault quite clearly differentiates (Foucault 1977a: 123, 138, 1977b: 200). Genealogy supplies apparently convincing analyses of historical changes in discursive practices, filled with examples drawn from the surface manifestations. The existence of a discourse is discerned inductively, and with enough ingenuity any text can be linked to a 'discourse'. For instance, having documented various Victorian texts which reported studies of the association of sugar with dental decay, Nettleton concludes that:

> Each of these studies with their various and often conflicting conclusions was an attempt to find the 'truth' about the relationship between sugar and caries. But there was a more fundamental truth which each of these studies has already presumed, namely the existence of mouths, teeth, sugar and disease. . . . In effect, arguments for and against [sugar's] value were all part of the same discourse.
>
> (Nettleton 1992: 81)

This is strictly Foucauldian: the rules of discursive formation provide the 'conditions of existence' of particular statements, which make it possible to say certain things and not others: the 'discourse' is inductively derived from the texts under study. But what precisely is happening here? The ontology requires that discourse is anonymous, dependent neither on human intent nor historical context, and cannot be reduced to the texts of specific 'authors' (Foucault 1977a: 121), yet genealogy concerns itself principally with texts, from which we 'uncover' the discourse. Freundlieb suggests (1994: 176) that behind such analysis is a 'hidden model of historical sociology' which links discursive practices to historical events (non-discursive practices) in precisely the way that Foucault rejected. Capitalism, industrial development, the physicality of the body, particular historical events or whatever form an unacknowledged backcloth which structures the analytical work of discerning the 'rules' of discursive formation.

In summary, it has been argued that Foucault's approach can 'rehabilitate' structuralist and functionalist kinds of analysis which de-emphasise agency, by rejecting 'sovereign' power and thus overcoming the determinism of such analyses (Silverman 1985). In this section I have suggested that when Foucault's ontology is scrutinised more closely, this resolution is actually rather less successful than has been argued, and depends on partial readings. On one hand, the ontology invokes the highly deterministic notion of rules of discursive formation, while on the other, genealogy may depend on authorial intent to a greater extent than is admitted. These tendencies towards determinism and humanism will be revisited in the next two sections.

FOUCAULT'S ONTOLOGY OF THE BODY

In his effort to avoid the 'liberal conception of individuals as unconstrained, creative essences' (Wickham 1986: 15), Foucault chose in his earlier work to de-privilege rationality and focus on the body as the site and target of power. As such, it also became the target of Foucault's methodology: genealogy, which he suggested is:

> a form of history which can account for the constitution of knowledges, discourses, domains of objects, etc. without having to make reference to a subject which is either transcendental in relation to the field of events or runs in its empty sameness throughout the course of history.
>
> (Foucault 1986: 59)

The problems of such an ontological re-focusing can be observed in the emergence of a 'sociology of the body' (Turner 1984, 1992; Nettleton 1995). By making the 'body' the new privileged object of a sociology, a new essentialism beckons, in which the body becomes the pre-existing focus of power's action, in place of a 'self', an 'individual' or an 'agent' (Wickham 1986). There is the potential for the Foucauldian body to become a romantic subject-substitute, continually buffeted by discourse, never able to self-actualise, doomed always to be the plaything of power/knowledge (Hacking 1986: 28). To avoid such essentialism, we need to be clear *which* body is the object of study. I would suggest four options.

1 The body is the physical body. For the strict Foucauldian, such a position is not acceptable. Foucault argues that power does not act directly on some biological entity (1976: x). Indeed, the concept of the biological body, the 'organism' or 'body-with-organs' (Deleuze and Guattari 1988: 158) is itself discursively constructed – by theology, by philosophy, by bio-medicine and other discourses.

2 It is some kind of 'natural body' overlaid with cultural values. This is an essentialist position, albeit one in which the essence's existence is determined phenomenologically, through 'experience', faith or 'common sense' (see, for example, Collins 1994). This position has been adopted in some post-structuralist feminisms, which while taking on board the perspective of the body as discursively constructed, wish at the same time to recognise the specific experience of sexual difference (McNay 1992: 36).

3 There is some kind of 'natural' body, but it is beyond discourse and thus unknowable. This avoids the tag of essentialism, but leaves us with a meaningless and pointless construct. As such, the 'sociology of the body' becomes the 'sociology of?'.

4 It is always already some kind of socially constructed body and it is 'impossible to know the materiality of the body outside its cultural significations' (McNay 1992: 30). While there are certain actions and gestures in physical space, certain states of mind within the brain, anything which can be called a unified 'body' is the creation of power/knowledge. This Foucauldian body – a 'body-*without*-organs' (Deleuze and Guattari 1984, 1988) – is a social body throughout.

Foucault himself seemed entirely unconcerned about whatever kind of material entity the body might be, and the way he wrote of the body implied that he often did not have in mind a conventional notion of the body at all (see, for example, Foucault 1977c: 169–70). For Foucault, the important thing was not the body itself, but that it was both realized in the play of power and also the site of possible transgressions or refusals of power (Game 1991: 45). Civilisation as the project of history relentlessly writes this body, seeking its total destruction by its transfiguration into a cultural object (Butler 1990: 129–30). This formulation reveals another aspect of the determinism of Foucault's ontology. Foucault's version of the body, despite his obvious political and personal inclinations to be on the side of those who are resistant

(Haber 1994), turns out to be 'totally imprinted by discourse' (Butler 1990), and 'passive and largely deprived of causal powers' (Lash 1991: 261–70). Ontologically, the model cannot analyse the conditions under which resistance to power becomes possible, why some people resist and others do not, and how resistance may be successful. And although the model may be a useful tool for analysis, it cannot be a catalyst for resistance (Haber 1994: 111): while resistance is always an aspect of power (Foucault 1980a: 142), to codify it is to vitiate it as resistance.

In summary, the ontology of Foucault's body leaves it passive. First, it cannot be allowed to be an agent: to provide it with such a capacity is to reintroduce the essentialism which Foucault wishes to deny. But second, and crucially, it is always already a cultural artifact which (referring back to the previous section) has a relation to the (non-discursive) body of history only through the anonymous discourse of power/knowledge. There is no way in this ontology for the non-discursive physical body to engage with the discursive body. Perhaps it is unsurprising that such an ontology of the body – once unpacked – seems inadequate to sociologists (Turner 1992: 57). Sociology has traditionally asked more of the body – for it to be an interface between different domains: biological and social, collective and individual, constrained and free (Bertholet 1991: 398).

FOUCAULT'S ONTOLOGY OF THE SELF

The later Foucault's work is noted for a turn from the body to 'the self' as its focus. As such, does the 'return of the subject' in the later Foucault reflect an about-turn, addressing the issue raised in the previous section? The ontological problem concerning resistance was one which Foucault was to acknowledge (often with great poignancy) in many later interviews (for example Martin 1988), and as he laboured to construct an ethics of the self, he wrote of individuals not as docile bodies but as reflexive, living, speaking beings (Foucault 1985: 7). The reflexive self theorised in volumes 2 and 3 of the *History of Sexuality* (*The Use of Pleasure* and *The Care of the Self*) contributes a more active notion of subjectivity, in place of the passive bodies of the earlier carceral model (McNay 1992: 49–50). A living, speaking, reflexive subjectivity implies the capacity to resist, and Foucault (1977c: 165) appeared to endorse Deleuze's theorising of a mechanism by which such an active subject may actively interpret and rewrite discourse and hence its own subjectivity (Lash 1991: 264–6). Although never explicitly revising his ontology, writing in 1982, he wondered whether perhaps:

I've insisted too much on the technology of domination and power. I am more and more interested in the interaction between oneself and others and in the technologies of individual domination, the history of how an individual acts upon himself, in the technology of the self.

(Foucault 1988: 19)

In this later writing, 'individual' and 'self' supplement the more usual 'subject' and 'body'; in his writing on the *History of Sexuality* (Foucault 1981, 1985, 1986, 1988) the move from concern with external technologies of power to technologies of the self is clear. Now, Foucault's project is with how we become 'desiring subjects'; in other words, how we articulate our bodies and desires within a subjectivity capable of reflection. 'Practices of the self' mark the engagement between discourses of the social and the individual, such that power is integral to the autonomous ordering of individuals' own lives (McNay 1992: 67). Foucault's genealogy of sexuality from ancient Greece, through early Christianity to the medieval and modern periods, explores different practices of the self and how these articulate with the discourses of the differing philosophical traditions. No longer is this described in terms of the imposition of discourse on passive bodies, but as a 'governmentality' in which technologies of domination articulate with technologies of the self, so as to:

permit individuals to effect by their own means or with the help of others a certain number of operations on their own bodies and souls, thoughts, conducts, and way of being, so as to transform themselves in order to attain a certain state of happiness, purity, wisdom, perfection or immortality.

(Foucault 1988: 18)

Personal identities thus emerge not as prior and privileged ontologically, but 'in a battlefield', in which difference and opposition are the means by which identity and the boundaries of others become discernible (Pizzorno 1992: 207). This is not unlike the formulation developed at the beginning of this paper in relation to the TF framework, and overcomes the criticism of Foucault's ontology which leaves individuals as passive and totally inscribed by discourse, for now it can be seen that reflexivity plays a crucial part in the process of subjectivity. Yet the ontological implications of Foucault's later position need further scrutiny, and three issues have been raised by critics.

First, as Pizzorno (1992) suggests, while we no longer have the liberal conception of subject as an individual bearer of interests and pursuer of ends:

> what stands opposed to power and ends up free or subjected (normalised) are acts, gestures, states of mind and body. Among them is to be found the *recalcitrant, resistant, unyielding material* that normalising power may fail to reduce.
>
> (1992: 207; my emphasis)

Wickham (1986) suggests that this implies an essentialising of resistance, pointing to the references in *Power/Knowledge* in which Foucault speaks of something which escapes power, which is an 'inverse energy', a 'discharge', 'energies and irreducibilities' (Foucault 1980a–d). Resistance is predicated upon this notion of something beyond and irreducible to discourse (Hoy 1986: 8), a position in apparent contradiction to all that has gone before concerning the relationship between discourse and the non-discursive.

Second, by emphasising the autonomy of the individual, within a governmentality which leads to a relativist 'art of existence' (that is, a reflexive and contextualised sense of what it means to be a self), Foucault's 'techniques of the self' are reduced to 'self-stylisations', failing to differentiate between 'practices that are merely "suggested" to the individual, and practices that are more or less "imposed" in so far as they are heavily laden with cultural sanctions and taboos' (McNay 1992: 74). Governmentality seems to offer such a degree of autonomy to the individual that it effectively shifts the balance from Foucault's earlier determinism concerning the 'rules' which determine which practices become discursive, to a relatively autonomous subjectivity.

Third, it was noted in the previous section that genealogy focuses for its raw material on texts. This becomes clearest in Foucault's final writings, on sexuality. Poster (1986) argues that, whereas in such works as *Discipline and Punish* Foucault could interpret Bentham's texts on the Panopticon in ways which turned the author's intentions on their heads (1986: 217), *The Care of the Self* (Vol. 3 of *The History of Sexuality*) is closer to a traditional history of ideas, relying heavily upon the intentional level of meaning and explicit phrases of 'key' textual accounts (for example, the writings of Plato or Marcus Aurelius). As such, Foucault leaves himself open to traditional criticisms concerning the justification of precisely which texts are 'key'. Both Poster (1986: 218) and Lois McNay (1992: 77–9) have subjected Foucault's efforts to interpret historical notions of sexuality, such as ancient Greek attitudes to sexual over-indulgence, to alternative explanations. 'Discourse' has become a moveable feast.

In summary, the shifts of emphasis in Foucault's ontology undermine most aspects of his earlier position concerning discourse and its relation to the non-discursive. The non-discursive 'residue' enables resistance to power/knowledge, no doubt providing a resource to the reflexive self as it is inscribed by discourse, while such subjects contribute to the generation of discourse through their texts. From what might be seen as an over-emphasis on determinism, we now find an over-emphasis on agency. Perhaps, as Rorty suggests, this was Foucault's dilemma, consequent on his twin aspirations – both to be a moral citizen concerned with the possibilities for resistance to power, and to refuse to be complicit with power by taking on its own vocabulary of essentialised subjects (Rorty 1992: 330–1). While his earlier work met the latter objective at the expense of the former, the re-introduction of a self privileges the former but makes his previous ontology untenable.

THE ONTOLOGY OF THE TF POSITION

These sections have been deconstructive of Foucault's ontology, with the intention of subsequently reconstructing a position which sustains a post-structuralist and post-humanist perspective, as outlined in the first few pages of this chapter. I will continue this effort now, looking at the TF in terms of the three areas under which I analysed Foucault's ontology.

Discourse, knowledge and power

From the TF perspective, there are no 'rules' of discursive formation. Texts become incorporated into particular framings through intertextual reading, and part of this process of framing entails the fabrication of particular patternings of intertextuality which we experience as subjectivity or sense-of-self. From time to time, these framings become 'differends' (Lyotard 1988) which are able – temporarily and locally – to deny contrary readings. This may be because of:

(a) some event of history (for example, political circumstances, economics, ageing or disease),
(b) the exertion of sovereign power, or
(c) the complicity of one or many for whom the *differend* links to history in ways which are pleasurable, advantageous or ethically attractive.

Because reading which ascribes meaning is necessarily a framing, it is thus a denial of difference, a moment when the intertext is refused. Power is thus not anonymous, it is located in the process of reading, although its effects work through texts, especially when these are framed in ways which become *differends*. Power may thus be coercive and/or a feature of this refusal of differentiation. Power is associated with knowledge, but 'knowledge' is simply one kind of *differend*.

The body

Bodies are not privileged in this ontology, nor are they are primary sites for the action of power. Bodies are cultural artifacts, fabricated both in the writing and reading of 'body texts', which will include the interpretation of aspects of spatial and temporal existence such as pain, pleasure, birth, ageing and death. As soon as one 'knows' one own or another's body, it has been written discursively; there can be no knowledge of a pre-social essential body, yet the epiphenomena of spatio-temporal existence are always rewriting the ways in which we know bodies. Anatomy, epidemiology, psychology, medical sociology and other body-texts frame bodies, often creating *differends* which know the body and exercise power over its reading.

The self

We actively engage in framing ourselves and others – discursively writing ourselves in relation to others and to history. Because all texts may be re-read, and it is reception rather than authorial intent which is relevant to sense-of-self, we are not subjects of discourse in a Foucauldian sense. While we are all potentially victims of the violence of the *differend*, through our own or through others' intertextual play, new possibilities continually open up for our sense of ourselves to 'become other' (Deleuze and Guattari 1988). Liberation (in this sense of becoming other) is thus not only possible, but is a continual feature of intertextual subjectivity. As such 'the other' is always important for our sense of who we are (Deleuze and Guattari 1988; Cixous 1990). The self, however, is also subject to history: to constraints and to threats (sovereign power).

The ontology of the TF position begins and ends with language, but not with language as something 'outside' of humans, but as achieved dialogically by humans, in engagement with others and in continual negotiation and misunderstanding. To see the potential application of the model in the deconstruction of textuality, I conclude with a brief example from the study of health and healing.

FRAMING THE TEXT: THE DISCHARGE

The following exchange is taken from fieldwork on surgery undertaken by the author (Fox 1992) and occurred between surgeon Mr D and patient Mr Y during a post-operative ward round. Even such a brief extract contains great richness in terms of the readings which the participants bring to the engagement.

> (*Mr D, the junior staff and the researcher gather round Mr Y's bed*)
> | | |
> |---|---|
> | Mr D | (*to patient, looking at chart*) Hallo Mr Y. Well we want to send you home, but I don't like that raised temperature. |
> | Patient Y | No. |
> | Mr D | 'I don't know what can be causing it. We've cultured the wound and there's no infection there. I just don't know what's causing it. . . . Are things ready for you to go home? |
> | Patient Y | Yes, my wife can come and collect me today. |
> | Mr D | Can you go to bed, and she can look after you? |
> | Patient Y | Yes. |
> | Mr D | I don't like that raised temperature. Phone your wife and you can go home now. |
> | Patient Y | Thank you very much. |

Of course, the number of texts which may be discerned in this engagement is potentially endless, because as readers we ourselves engage intertextually and thus productively with this text (Fox 1995), and there can be no 'final' or ultimately correct reading. Amongst others, we might identify:

(a) the body of the patient,
(b) the context of the surgical ward, and the operation on Mr Y,
(c) surgery as a discipline/skill/profession,
(d) Mr D's professional occupation,
(e) Mr Y's history as a patient, including the chart held by Mr D,
(f) Mr Y's biography, and his home and life outside the hospital.

Some of these are literally texts, while others are 'social' or 'body' texts, and the impact of each will depend on its framing. However, the deconstruction is not wholly unwieldy, as what are of interest are those frames which mediate the power relations of the encounter; in other words, those which serve as *differends*, violently disrupting the free flow of intertextuality, and working at a text's frame, at the delimitation of a text or where two or more texts collide.

What might be the *differends* here: the framings which write Mr Y and Mr D, silencing other voices, other textualities? There is the ward, and there is the bed which Mr Y is sitting upon while Mr D and the rest of us stand over him. There is bio-medicine, with its definitions and mystique of language. But perhaps the framing which is of greatest rhetorical use here is Mr Y's chart, on which is inscribed a text of his body in terms of temperature, heart rate, etc. The chart has a very literal frame, in that it covers the period of Mr Y's hospitalisation. Beyond this temporal frame past and future cease to have any relevance. And it has a second metaphorical frame in its concerns with bio-medically defined vital signs.

Mr D holds the chart, he is in control of it and Mr Y does not get to see it. Mr D uses the chart's *frame* in *framing* the opening remarks, to mark out his authority over Mr Y's disposal. The chart frames Mr Y in terms of time and the signs recorded there. Nothing outside the frame of the chart is to be considered now, and the chart's bio-medical framing sets the parameters within which the decision is to be. Anything which is beyond the chart is excluded, Mr Y is written by the chart, he is the chart.

While this *differend* supplies Mr D's control of the situation, this framing is provisional and Mr D admits this himself, because the chart reveals something disturbing about Mr Y: he has a raised temperature, a possible complication which will need to be resolved before discharge. Mr D *doesn't like* this raised temperature. Why? First, because it means Mr Y *is not fit*, not fit for discharge. Second (and he uses the identical phrase a second time), Mr D doesn't like it because it means Mr Y *does not fit* the framing which he wants to impose, of Mr Y as healed, an ex-patient, ready for discharge.

But Mr D wants this annoying temperature not to fit, to be excluded from his decision-making. So he must victimise it, creating a new *differend* to exclude it. Raised temperatures are things patients have, but Mr Y (Mr D wishes to demonstrate) is a non-patient, a success of surgery, he should have none of the attributes of a patient. To construct the *differend*, Mr D tests the limits of the text which is Mr Y and his raised temperature: the temperature is nothing to do with the operation ('there's no infection'), it is irrelevant ('I just don't know what's causing it'), Mr Y is ready to go home, his wife is ready to take him away, he will continue his recuperation at home, he is physically capable of action ('phone your wife'). Mr D disallows the raised temperature any rights to define Mr Y. Mr Y is written as an ex-patient; no doubt in time, he will be written up.

FINAL FRAME: AFTER FOUCAULT?

Within the TF perspective, history provides the raw material for the endless play of difference which is intertextuality. At the same time, at least in part, history is also the product of intertextuality. Bodies and selves are written and read, as the patterns of intensity of the texts which impinge on them wax and wane. To appropriate a maxim from Marx, we write history, but not in texts of our own choosing. The framing of texts which enables them to 'make sense' sometimes leads to the creation of victims: those who are unable to speak in the face of the *differend*. But the same process of framing provides the possibility of resistance, for a subjectivity which can 'become other', which is not constrained by rules of discursive formation. There are signs, and more signs, and then more . . . .

Foucault's frame of reference rewrites human subjects in ways which challenge humanist understandings of self and others. Perhaps it is not surprising that the ontology is ambiguous and contradictory; that is a feature of any intertextual enterprise which seeks to persuade. The TF position has its own *differend* and may be subjected to deconstruction. In that sense, there is nothing 'after' Foucault: all positions are read in a space which is atemporal and has no spatial limits, they are defined by the play of differences from each other. They depend on each other (as postmodernism relies on modernism so as to have an object of critique), and none is right or wrong. If one falls out of favour, that perhaps is good enough reason to seek its reinstatement. If another becomes dominant, perhaps that is enough reason to wish to resist the violence of its *differend*.

REFERENCES

Armstrong, D. (1983) *The Political Anatomy of the Body*, Cambridge: Cambridge University Press.

Barthes, R. (1977) *Image–Music–Text*, Glasgow: Collins Fontana.

Bertholet, J.M. (1991) 'Sociological discourse and the body', in M. Featherstone, M. Hepworth and B. Turner (eds) *The Body: Social Process and Cultural Theory*, London: Sage.

Brown, B. and Cousins, M. (1986) 'The linguistic fault: the case of Foucault's archaeology', in M. Gane (ed.) *Towards a Critique of Foucault*, London: Routledge and Kegan Paul.

Butler, J. (1990) *Gender Trouble: Feminism and the Subversion of Identity*, London: Routledge.

Cixous, H. (1990) 'The laugh of the Medusa', in R. Walder (ed.) *Literature in the Modern World: Critical Essays and Documents*, Oxford: Oxford University Press.

Collins, H. (1994) 'Dissecting surgery: forms of life depersonalized', *Social Studies of Science*, 24, 2: 311–34.

Deleuze, G. and Guattari, F. (1984) *Anti-Oedipus: Capitalism and Schizophrenia*, London: Athlone.

Deleuze, G. and Guattari, F. (1988) *A Thousand Plateaus*, London: Athlone.

Derrida, J. (1987) *The Truth in Painting*, Chicago: University of Chicago Press.

Donnelly, M. (1986) 'Foucault's genealogy of the human sciences', in M. Gane (ed.) *Towards a Critique of Foucault*, London: Routledge and Kegan Paul.

Dreyfus, H.L. and Rabinow, P. (1982) *Michel Foucault: Beyond Structuralism and Hermeneutics*, Chicago: University of Chicago Press.

Foucault, M. (1974) *The Archaeology of Knowledge*, London: Tavistock.

Foucault, M. (1976) *Birth of the Clinic. An Archaeology of Medical Perception*, London: Tavistock.

Foucault, M. (1977a) 'What is an author?', in D.F. Bouchard (ed.) *Language, Counter-Memory, Practice*, Oxford: Blackwell.

Foucault, M. (1977b) 'History of systems of thought', in D.F. Bouchard (ed.) *Language, Counter-Memory, Practice*, Oxford: Blackwell.

Foucault, M. (1977c) 'Theatrum Philosophicum', in D.F. Bouchard (ed.) *Language, Counter-Memory, Practice*, Oxford: Blackwell.

Foucault, M. (1979) *Discipline and Punish: The Birth of the Prison*, Harmondsworth: Peregrine.

Foucault, M. (1980a) 'The eye of power', in C. Gordon (ed.) *Power/Knowledge*, Brighton: Harvester Press.

Foucault, M. (1980b) 'Truth and power', in C. Gordon (ed.) *Power/Knowledge*, Brighton: Harvester Press.

Foucault, M. (1980c) 'Two lectures', in C. Gordon (ed.) *Power/Knowledge*, Brighton: Harvester Press.

Foucault, M. (1980d) 'The confession of the flesh', in C. Gordon (ed.) *Power/Knowledge*, Brighton: Harvester Press.

Foucault, M. (1981) *The History of Sexuality, Vol. 1: An Introduction*, Harmondsworth: Penguin.

Foucault, M. (1985) *The Use of Pleasure (Vol. 2 of the History of Sexuality)*, New York: Pantheon.

Foucault, M. (1986) *The Care of the Self (Vol. 3 of the History of Sexuality)*, New York: Pantheon.

Foucault, M. (1988) 'Technologies of the self', in L.H. Martin, H. Gutman and P.H. Hutton (eds) *Technologies of the Self: A Seminar with Michel Foucault*, London: Tavistock.

Fox, N.J. (1992) *The Social Meaning of Surgery*, Buckingham: Open University Press.

Fox, N.J. (1993) *Postmodernism, Sociology and Health*, Buckingham: Open University Press.

Fox, N.J. (1995) 'Intertextuality and the writing of social research', *Electronic Journal of Sociology* 1, 3: no page numbers.

Freundlieb, D. (1994) 'Foucault's theory of discourse and human agency', in C. Jones and R. Porter (eds) *Reassessing Foucault: Power, Medicine and the Body*, London: Routledge.

Game, A. (1991) *Undoing the Social: Towards a Deconstructive Sociology*, Buckingham: Open University Press.

Haber, H. (1994) *Beyond Postmodern Politics: Lyotard, Rorty, Foucault*, London: Routledge.

Hacking, I. (1986) 'The archaeology of Foucault', in D.C. Hoy (ed.) *Foucault: A Critical Reader*, Oxford: Blackwell.

Hoy, D.C. (1986) 'Introduction', in D.C. Hoy (ed.) *Foucault: A Critical Reader*, Oxford: Blackwell.

Lash, S. (1991), 'Genealogy and the body: Foucault/Deleuze/Nietzsche', in M. Featherstone, M. Hepworth and B.S. Turner (eds) *The Body: Social Process and Cultural Theory*, London: Sage.

Lupton, D. (1994) *Medicine as Culture: Illness, Disease and the Body in Western Societies*, London: Sage.

Lyotard, J. (1988) *The Differend: Phrases in Dispute*, Minneapolis: University of Minnesota Press.

McNay, L. (1992) *Foucault and Feminism: Power, Gender and the Self*, Oxford: Polity.

Martin, R. (1988) 'Truth, power, self: an interview with Michel Foucault', in L.H. Martin, H. Gutman and P.H. Hutton (eds) *Technologies of the Self: A Seminar with Michel Foucault*, London: Tavistock.

Nettleton, S. (1992) *Power, Pain and Dentistry*, Buckingham: Open University Press.

Nettleton, S. (1995) *The Sociology of Health and Illness*, Cambridge: Polity.

Pizzorno, A. (1992) 'Foucault and the liberal view of the individual', in T.J. Armstrong (ed.) *Michel Foucault, Philosopher*, New York: Harvester Wheatsheaf.

Poster, M. (1986) 'Foucault and the tyranny of Greece', in D.C. Hoy (ed.) *Foucault: A Critical Reader*, Oxford: Blackwell.

Rorty, R. (1992) 'Moral identity and private autonomy', in T.J. Armstrong (ed.) *Michel Foucault, Philosopher*, New York: Harvester Wheatsheaf.

Silverman, D. (1985) *Qualitative Methodology and Sociology*, Aldershot: Gower.

Smart, B. (1985) *Michel Foucault*, London: Tavistock.

Turner, B. (1984) *The Body and Society: Explorations in Social Theory*, Oxford: Blackwell.

Turner, B. (1992) *Regulating Bodies: Essays in Medical Sociology*, London: Routledge.

Valverde, M. (1991) 'As if subjects exist; analysing social discourses', *Canadian Review of Anthropology and Sociology*, 28, 2: 173–87.

Wickham, G. (1986) 'Power and power analysis: beyond Foucault?', in M. Gane (ed.) *Towards a Critique of Foucault*, London: Routledge.

Part II

Discourses of health and medicine

Chapter 3

Mental health, criminality and the human sciences

David McCallum

INTRODUCTION: LAW AND PSYCHIATRY

Thirty years after its publication, Michel Foucault's *Madness and Civilization* still provokes debate among historians. It is 'a beautiful book', a set of 'over-simplifications' flying in the face of empirical evidence, and a new model for writing the history of culture (Foucault 1965; Midelfort 1980; O'Brien 1989). A recent survey of the book's reception claimed that there had been no real test of the fruitfulness of Foucault's 'complex interpretive framework', and so for some his status as a historian of madness must remain an open question (Gutting 1994). Foucault's writings have been a source of 'irritation' for historians, often because his work has raised difficult questions about the politics of history-writing and the role of the intellectual. He addressed some of these criticisms in 'Questions of method' (Foucault 1991) and other places where he attempted to answer the claim that his work provided no encompassing explanatory framework. He said that his critics complained of no structure in his work: 'no infra- or superstructure, no Malthusian cycle, no opposition between state and civil society: none of these schemas which have bolstered historians' operations, explicitly or implicitly, for the past hundred or hundred and fifty years' (Foucault 1991: 85). The debates specifically on the history of madness continue, despite the fact that the abridged English translation still makes Foucault's original *Histoire de la folie* something of an 'unknown book' to English readers (Gordon 1990).

While for some the jury might be still out on 'Foucault the historian', there ought to be less reluctance to acknowledge the contribution which Foucault, and those influenced by his work, have made to the method of enquiry he described as 'histories of the present' – the use of historical investigation for the purposes of diagnosing problems in the here and now. A major field of interest to Foucault concerned the contemporary functioning of the penal system, the mental health system and other dispersed sets of institutional mechanisms of governing, as a way of seeking to problematise the forms in which freedom is exercised in modern liberal societies (Burchell 1993). In this sense, Foucault's work has encouraged new approaches to old questions largely as a consequence of the conceptual 'toolbox' he developed through his own historical enquiries. So rather than providing 'schemas' and closures, the implied intellectual invitation is to take up his methods of enquiry as a way of charting new territories and formulating questions in different sorts of ways. His works on the asylum and the prison, posed in terms of disciplinary techniques, ought to stand as exemplary points of departure on methodological grounds, as well as on the grounds of the sheer weight of the historiography. His use of historical investigation is as a philosopher seeking to elucidate questions of the present rather than the professional historian providing an empirically sound record of the past. Foucault sought to make more limited claims about the role of the intellectual by providing the 'instruments of analysis . . . a topological and geological survey of the battlefield' (Foucault 1980; Weeks 1982), and to use history as an aid to making maps of as yet unexplored regions of human affairs (Deleuze 1993).

Much of the conventional historical work on criminality and madness consists of discrete works charting the internal dynamics of institutional development of these two domains. Foucault's interventions into law and psychiatry have provided a theoretical warrant to problematise such fields in ways which emphasise their convergences and interrelations. As he has shown, the complex interdependencies in the contemporary operation of law and psychiatry followed from the transformation of criminal responsibility within early nineteenth-century European penal law, where increasingly the intelligibility of a criminal act came to be referenced against the character and antecedents of the individual. Foucault wrote:

> The more psychologically determined an act is found to be, the more its author can be considered legally responsible. The more the act is, so to speak, gratuitous and undetermined, the more it will tend to be excused. A paradox, then: the legal freedom of a subject is proven by the fact that his act is seen to be necessary, determined; his lack of responsibility proven by the fact that his act is seen to be unnecessary.
> (Foucault 1988: 140)

The reciprocal functionality of law and psychiatry made it possible, later in the century, to establish the determination of not just the great and monstrous crime but also everyday minor infractions and common delinquency, along an increasingly diverse psychological and psychiatric register. As conceptions of insanity and mental illness shifted, the psychiatric and criminological continuum could allow for an almost infinite proliferation of psycho-medical conditions and categories of person. The recognition of this historical collaboration of law and psychiatry, and the implications of the 'psychiatrization of criminal danger' (1988: 125), is critical to an understanding of the evolution of psychological and psychiatric categories and their social functioning in the present. By themselves, neither the conventional psychiatric histories nor the more dispersed histories of penal law and criminality are helpful in formulating these perspectives. Categories of person do not emerge into the present by means of a continuous line of development traceable within the histories of either psychiatry or criminality, but rather are constituted at the intersection of both domains.

This chapter is concerned to examine the synergism of the psycho-medical concept of personality disorder and calculations of dangerousness. The language and conceptual terrain of personality disorder have entered into the routines of calculating and administering 'problem' groups in social work, the magistrates' courts, the mental health system, and cases of horrific crime. Attention has been given in psychiatric, psychological and legal studies literature to the problem of dangerousness, and the interrelations between the criminal justice and mental health systems in their management (Floud and Young 1981; Reid 1985; Kissane 1990; Parker 1991). One underlying premise is that law and medicine simply have different interests in the matter: the doctor being concerned with diagnosis and treatment, the courts with the relationship between a person and a particular act (O'Sullivan 1981: 2). Yet the debates have left this field of 'personhood' quite problematic. Psychiatric expertise in Australia has claimed that recent cases in law have revealed a 'fundamental inability to define conceptual boundaries' (Glaser 1994: 115–16). Some legal expertise has argued the need for a more 'flexible' legal theory in order to allow for the confinement of those considered to be dangerous, rather than resorting to 'fictions' about a person's psychiatric condition (Williams 1990: 182). Whether or not personality disorder is a mental illness is an ongoing source of controversy between the two sectors (American Psychiatric Association 1982; Campbell 1988: 15ff). There has been no authoritative and generally accepted medical definition of what constitutes 'disease of the mind' (Bartholomew and Milte 1976: 451); diagnosis of mental illness lacks reliability, and psychiatry is generally unable to predict dangerousness with any great precision (Cocozza and Steadman 1976; Fairall 1993).

The distinctiveness of the concept of personality was emphasised in a recent debate in Victoria over whether to change the Mental Health Act to classify persons with an anti-social personality disorder (Law Reform Commission of Victoria 1990). Complaints over possible breaches of mental health rights came from members of the psychiatric profession, from legal expertise, and from health consumer groups. Glaser (1990) claimed that to exclude personality disorder from mental health provisions was in keeping with the definitions of 'key concepts', and 'the development of *psychological* concepts such as "personality" and "personality disorder"' (emphasis added):

> 'Personality' simply refers to a person's characteristic way of functioning psychologically: in the same way that people may be fat, thin or bald, so various individuals may be described as shy, friendly or sensitive. A 'personality disorder' differs from a 'normal' personality only as a matter of degree. Thus, we all do morally and socially 'bad' things some of the time; and a person with an 'anti-social personality disorder' is just somewhat more 'bad' than the rest of the community. She or he lies, cheats, has trouble with the police, is involved in multiple unstable relationships and has a poor work record.
>
> (Glaser 1990: 114)

Personality, Glaser argued, referred to a way of functioning psychologically since childhood. In contrast, mental illness resulted in a qualitative change in personality, involving a fairly sudden change in behaviour (1990: 114). Although the Mental Health Act did not define what mental illness was, it did set out the conditions to be satisfied before a mentally ill person can be involuntarily admitted to a hospital. On this point, psychiatry established the justification for excluding personality disorder. Section 8(2) of the Act lists anti-social personality disorder alongside instances of 'social and political deviance' which ought not to be used to justify involuntary detention: expressing certain political beliefs, engaging in unusual forms of sexual activity or being intellectually disabled. Because of their social position, some persons were also more likely to be defined as having an anti-social personality than others. In this view, an attempt to assert that 'persistent badness' was an illness which must be treated against a person's will constituted a danger to civil liberties and was antithetical to a free society (Glaser 1990: 115–16).

As an alternative point of departure, it is proposed to examine the language and conceptual terrain of personality disorder in terms of the way in which language carves out new domains of existence and new spaces for the play of public powers. This is to look at language as an instrument for producing new forms of thought about persons, and new ways of calculating those very areas of human affairs which need to be managed and governed. It is to suggest that language as an 'intellectual technology' acts over time to produce knowledges of particular types of existence and categories of person, in order to seek to manage individuals and govern populations (Miller and Rose 1988, 1990). The category of personality disorder can be seen in precisely these terms. How did the category come about; how do distinctions and specificities in terminology such as 'personality' come into being? Or rather, how has it become possible to 'think' the problem of dangerousness and violation of social order within the psycho-medical category of personality disorder? Let me make some initial remarks on the history of the distinctions between lunatics, idiots and criminals and their common institutional location, before moving on to examining the techniques for calculating personality as a new interior space of individuality.

SEPARATING PRACTICES: TECHNIQUES OF CALCULATION

The distinction in law between lunatics and idiots existed in old English common law. A jury of twelve might find a person to be *purus idiota* in which case 'the profits of his lands, and the custody of his person' might be granted by the King to a person who had interest enough to obtain them (Blackstone 1972: 292). Similarly, the method of proving a person to be *non compos mentis* (a lunatic) was undertaken by the Lord Chancellor by special authority of the King, who would grant a commission of enquiry into a party's state of mind and, if the party was found *non compos*, would 'commit' his care along with an allowance to some friend who would then be called his 'committee'. These procedures followed historically from the repeal of the Witchcraft Acts in 1736, as well as various certification processes brought into being to protect the sane from wrongful detention. The safeguards against misuses of detention of the wealthy later extended to paupers. They were a development of an older royal prerogative for the Crown to act as guardian of idiots and warden of their estates in return for maintaining the idiot, which was formalised in early English statutes in the fourteenth century and later delegated to the Lord Chancellor and the Court of Chancery. These same powers were entrusted to Governor Phillip in his second Commission (Historical Records of Australia 1914: 4). For persons of substance, the process of enquiry *de lunatico inquirendo* continued until the Lunacy Act of 1878 created the Office of Master of Lunacy to manage the estates of insane persons.

The Australian psychiatric historian C.J. Cummins writes that early in the colony there was only a fine distinction between lunacy and 'social incompatibility' – the gaol was the common repository for both classes (Cummins 1967: 11). Housed initially with convicts in Parramatta gaol, lunatics drew the sympathy of Governor Macquarie, who then in 1811 allotted some farm buildings at Castle Hill for use as an asylum. Later, Governor Darling authorised the use of the court house at Liverpool and Hyde Park barracks for lunatics, after the Castle Hill site was reallocated for church use. From 1838 a new asylum at Tarban Creek was established with Joseph Digby as lay superintendent, beginning, Cummins announces, 'an era of psychiatry in Australia' (1967: 15). There followed a ten-year episode of conflict and bitterness between lay superintendent and medical officer which ended with a Committee of Inquiry recommendation that the asylum be headed by a 'medical man'. Cummins shows that the moves to formalise admission procedures requiring a medical certificate were instigated by the lay-superintendent Digby, who supposedly was acting on the basis of his knowledge of the English Act of 1828 which he had experienced while working at St Luke's asylum in London.

The original Female Factory at Parramatta in Sydney, established under Macquarie in 1821, was converted into an asylum for housing 'chronic and deteriorated patients', the first instance of separate accommodation being established for a specific group within the lunatic population. Cummins describes Parramatta as a 'benevolent asylum remarkably similar in purpose and content to an English workhouse' (1967: 21), which admitted, besides the 'harmless chronic dement', destitute persons suffering from a range of chronic diseases. The criminally insane were also housed at Tarban Creek until 1861 when a special asylum was erected in the grounds of Parramatta (1967: 25). Gaols continued to be used as a means of confining the 'wandering lunatic' and the 'vagrant' especially in rural areas, for convenience and to avoid admission to the asylum. Cummins claims the gaols thus acted as 'reception houses' for doubtful cases or for patients with acute episodes.

The first legislation on lunacy was the New South Wales Dangerous Lunatics Act of 1843, making provision for the 'safe custody of and prevention of offences by persons dangerously insane and for the care and maintenance of persons of unsound mind'. It provided the mechanism whereby the Governor could direct criminals who became insane, or insane persons committed for trial, or persons acquitted on the grounds of insanity, to a lunatic asylum. The latter group became known as 'governor's pleasure' inmates. The legislation also introduced a system of dual certification as part of the committal of the insane, a system which remained substantially intact until the provisions were altered in the 1958 Mental Health Act. At the time, a successful legal action against the lay superintendent for illegal confinement, brought by a certain Captain Hyndman (Coppe 1986), accelerated the first lunacy law through the Legislative Council giving the doctor control of the asylum.

Much of traditional Australian medical historiography is consistent with Cummins's view that the 'birth of psychiatry' can be located at the point of establishing the asylum, or at least when the medical man begins to take charge of the asylum during the 1840s in Australia. It is back there, to the half-light of the old asylum, that psychiatry is able to trace the continuous line of descent of modern categories such as the 'mentally ill'. One psychiatric historian talks of the 'torch of psychological insight' as a tool to retrospectively discover the mentally ill behind the lunatic of old (Bostock 1968: 18). Although the record of the sick in hospital in 1788 made no mention of nervous disorder, the 'paucity of information . . . is explicable under the hard living conditions of frontier life . . . there was neither time nor opportunity for records' (1969: 19). Similarly, in his history of 'mental health services' in Western Australia, A.S. Ellis claims that 'from the beginning the mentally ill were there' (Ellis 1983: 2). And in a recent summary of the historical research in psychiatry, Dax shows that 'psychiatric services in both New Zealand and Australia had their beginning in the gaols' (Dax 1981: 258). The point about these histories is that they tend to assume an a priori existence of madness, independently of its historically specific forms of calculation. The continuing figure of the 'mentally ill' forms part of a grid of modern psychological and psychiatric knowledges of persons which is then superimposed onto the past (Minson 1985: 207).

In contrast to these histories, the social history of madness focuses on the events which helped to determine the construction of the categories themselves. For example, conflict over the definition of categories of persons and professional jurisdictions is to be found in the close institutional connections in the nineteenth century between law and medicine, criminality and madness, the prison and the asylum. The modern dualism of the 'bad or mad' is able to be traced to common institutional sites for the disposal of these two categories of person (Garton 1982). Evidence brought from magistrates' courts and police lock-ups indicates a shift in incarceration practices (favouring the asylum over the prison) between the nineteenth and twentieth centuries, and a concomitant extension of mental health services over the whole of the population. By the mid-twentieth century, by virtue of this 'medicalisation', psychiatry came to supervise a range of phenomena known as 'psycho-pathological' that previously had been seen as moral and criminal problems (1982: 89).

These manoeuvres in social history give a warrant to investigate how categories of person were produced according to certain historical contingencies and specific knowledges and techniques of administration, rather than as a consequence of practices already defined as essentially 'law' or 'medicine', or in terms of given sets of oppositions such as the 'bad or mad'. It becomes possible to look more directly at the diversity of techniques deployed in calculating these different categories of person. A focus on techniques of calculation brings to the fore the question of how individuals come to be known and categorised, as acts of population management; that is, how the management of problem groups entails a kind of power in the form of applied knowledge, which produces certain kinds of persons and subjects.

Some recent historical work on personality and personality disorder provide some useful points of departure on the question of techniques of calculation. The Sydney psychiatrist John Ellard, in his provocatively titled *Some Rules for Killing People* (1989), has traced the early attempts towards formulating a taxonomy of psychiatric illness in the writings of Thomas Sydenham and Thomas Arnold at the end of the eighteenth century, in order to explain some of the 'confusions' in law and psychiatry. Ellard saw in the modern term 'anti-social personality disorder' a confusion of medicine and morals, the insane and the 'vicious', whose origins lay in a 'fundamental confusion' about the meaning of insanity in these founding texts (Ellard 1989: 119). Arnold's *Observations on the Nature, Kinds, Causes and Prevention of Insanity*, published in 1806, devised a notion of insanity which was supposed to exclude 'all but the really insane'; merely because certain persons were 'under the influence of strong, or even habitual passions . . . I reckon such persons vicious, but not insane', Arnold said. One had to be insane first, on definite criteria, and only then could certain vice-ridden behaviour be considered in assigning persons to a particular classification of insanity. Ellard's point is that Arnold's seemingly unambiguous distinction between insanity and viciousness was outlived by the category of the 'morally insane'. The confusion was further perpetuated in Pritchard's schema of 1837, where moral insanity became:

> a form of mental derangement, in which the intellectual faculties appear to have sustained little or no injury while the disorder is manifested principally alone, in the state of the feelings, tempers or habits.
>
> (Pritchard, cited in Ellard 1989: 121)

In 1844, Woodward said that moral insanity could be distinguished from mere depravity because it was always preceded or accompanied by 'some diseased function of organs' so subtle it could be detected by a psychiatrist but not by a court or jury. Ellard argued that this form of insanity 'existed only in the psychiatrist's imagination' (1989: 125). From Pritchard to the present day, the distinction between insanity and wickedness was lost in the successive confusion of medicine and morals: Issac Ray's 'moral mania' (1871), Spitzka's 'moral imbecility' (1887), Koch's 'psychopathic personality' (1891), Cleckley's 'psychopath' (1941), Bowlby's 'moral defective' (1949) and finally the *Diagnostic and Statistical Manual*'s 'sociopathic personality disturbance' (1952). As Ellard notes:

> The wheel has turned full circle; we are back with Pritchard, but not exactly. Whereas Pritchard's disorder was a derangement of the moral faculty, an entity in one's head, the DSM-III [*Diagnostic and Statistical Manual*, 3rd edn] disorder is of the traits. Traits are not entirely in one's head; they are 'enduring patterns of perceiving, relating to and thinking about the environment and oneself'. They are processes and not entities, factors rather than faculties. But only just.
>
> (1989: 129)

For Ellard, the 'psychopath' has become a household word because it retained the status of both explanation and cause. Why has a man done such terrible things? Because he is a psychopath. How do you know he is a psychopath? Because he has done these terrible things. In the end, the description of an anti-social personality disorder is essentially that of a 'hoodlum from a poor and disadvantaged family', a judgement arising from the customs and prejudices of a particular group from which psychiatrists are themselves drawn and who therefore fail to see this incongruity (1989: 130–1).

Ellard's account attempts to explain the current weaknesses of psychiatry as a weakness in scientific activity – by its failure to separate medicine from morals. Thus, current uncertainties of meaning and breaches of scientific convention can be traced to fundamental confusions reproduced over time in psychiatric texts, as science struggled to know its object independently of social and political strictures. Ellard's use of the older term 'moral insanity' was the starting point back into the history of what for him was a pseudo-science, in as much as it merely paralleled the narrow outlook and social position of psychiatric practitioners and theorists. His work assumes the continuous figure of the 'morally insane' through to the modern period, as psychiatry sought to clarify its categories. Ellard's account would support current legal and psychiatric opinion against changing mental health legislation in a way which would redefine a person by the use of psychiatric categories. We might recall Williams's argument, for example, that to advance a case for legal reform on the basis that 'medical facts' will be altered to conform to the will of legislators amounted to a perversion of scientific validation techniques and knowledge (Williams 1990). And similarly, Glaser declared that changing the Mental Health Act to incarcerate the dangerous was an attempt by the state to 'massively shift the power/knowledge balance in its favour' by attempting to redefine the boundaries of scientific knowledge for 'purely political purposes' (Glaser 1994: 46). Of course, this is not the epistemological scepticism of psychiatric knowledge evinced so clearly in Ellard's account. But nevertheless, all these accounts share a common assumption – that different categories of mental illness and disorder exist prior to, and independently of, their historically specific means of calculation.

The taken-for-grantedness of these categories is questioned in part by research which focuses more directly on the concept of personality and how it emerged from the activities of experimental psychology in the early part of the twentieth century. Danziger (1990) gives an account of how the concept of personality grew out of personality studies in psychology, in response to the limited grasp of intelligence testing on a broader range of qualities, such as leadership and assertiveness. Danziger points to the realisation among research psychologists in the US during the 1920s that the factor of intelligence was only one of the determinants of real-life performance, to which could be added character, personality, will, attitude and so on.

He illustrates how personality as a psychological/administrative category came into existence alongside the invention of the personality test itself. According to Danziger, personality as an object of research relied first on an 'additive' model of the person, whereby the contents of individuality can be given a numerical value, and second on the development of this numerical structure to refer to something which existed to some measurable amount across situations and persons, such as the possession of 'ascendance' or 'introversion'. As he explains, performances on personality tests were taken to reflect inherent properties revealed in the task of doing the test:

> the fundamental psychological meanings and reference of the empirical data were constituted by an interpretive construction that was not derived from those data but preceded their collection.
>
> (1990: 161)

Danziger claims that personality tests transformed a set of language terms such as 'dependence' into unambiguous properties of the natural world which could be investigated as a physicist might investigate electrical resistance. What this amounted to, for Danziger, was 'a masquerade in which categories generated by a very specific social order were held to represent an ahistorical natural order' (1990: 162). His work then explores the cultural preconceptions and interests of groups who were responsible for the development of the tests. The main strength of his analysis, however, for present purposes, is his account of the contribution by psychology to the production of personality as a calculable space, and to the new tools of calculation and the raft of statistical laws which emerged from the tests. Indeed, it is possible to argue from his evidence that personality itself was formed as a governable space hand in glove with the appearance of this object in the 'data' themselves (Hacking 1986).

This is to suggest, then, that conceptions of individuality framed around personality and its calculable properties may be understood as being not simply the result of the evolution of psychological concepts (Glaser), or of the residue of fundamental historical confusions of knowledge (Ellard), or of the effect of the limits of language to represent the empirical realities of the natural world (Danziger). These perspectives on knowledge and power do seem to imply that it is possible to conceive of psychiatric and psychological knowledges as potentially free of and unsullied by the effects of power. Instead, the problematising of personality might be understood as part of a 'history of political technologies of individuality'; of an analysis of the shifting forms in which 'political power has come to bear upon subjects, and has sought to understand them and govern them' (Rose 1990: 217). The emphasis is on the positive and productive effects of power, as distinct from a crushing of truths or the repression of rights.

There is reason to examine further the historical specificity of the means of calculating different categories and types of persons. Categories of person are the product of the available tools and techniques for knowing. So rather than personality disorder appearing as a problem which must be administered *by* government, it comes to be understood instead as an *effect of* techniques which seek to understand individuals and govern them. Personality is produced as a surface upon which the need to define the 'antecedents' of the individual in order to properly manage them is impressed. Personality becomes an artifact of government.

SEPARATING PERSONALITY

The first half of the twentieth century saw the gradual separation, both administratively and geographically, of an aggregate population into the mentally ill on the one hand, and the mentally defective and mentally deficient on the other. Such a separation is the main point of reference in documenting the circumstances of the emergence of personality disorder. The history of this separation parallels the history of psychology itself and the new tools which psychology either inherited, transformed or invented to bring human behaviour into the field of the calculable.

Long-standing distinctions between 'lunaticks and ideots' which had been brought over from England in Governor Phillip's letters of commission were temporal distinctions dependent on the permanency and the degree of a person's infirmity, which in turn had various administrative and legal consequences (Historical Records of Australia 1914), although we know these groups would routinely share institutional space for the next two hundred years. Much the same administrative, legislative and institutional arrangements for the mentally ill and the mentally defective or deficient were in place in the middle of the twentieth century. But the primary separation, beginning in the latter half of the nineteenth century, and gaining momentum in the early decades of the twentieth century, was not of lunatics and idiots, not of mental defectives from the mentally ill, but rather of acute and chronic inmates who previously shared space within the old lunatic asylum but who now found themselves in separate accommodation. The acute patients occupied the newly named 'acute mental hospitals' while the chronic and hopeless cases were farmed out to peripheral institutions. The chronic and hopeless were a loose aggregate of 'epileptics, congenital imbeciles, general paralytics, paranoiacs, and senile dements' (Victoria, Inspector-General of Insane, *Annual Report* 1915: 37), which attracted little practical interest for medicine as there was little it could do in terms of treatment, compared with the more interesting and prestigious acute patients. The chronics were often also less valuable in a strict economic sense because many could not perform work in the asylum. Their administrative separation from the mental hospital and from a strict medical gaze was underpinned by the increasing attention afforded them as suitable objects of education and training.

At first, moral insanity and moral imbecility fell fairly comfortably within the overall aggregate of lunatics and idiots, and insanity and imbecility, separated from each other by the same temporal distinctions that separated insanity from idiocy. Although it was clear that moral insanity and moral imbecility had the added distinction of criminal or immoral propensities, it was equally clear that the penal system was not the appropriate place to hold these persons:

> The moral insanity and moral imbecility here spoken of are peculiar mental affections, whose existence is proved beyond doubt. Moral imbecility is a congenital inability to distinguish between right and wrong, and to be influenced by punishment. It does not often endure to adult life, but is frequent in children. . . . The morally insane are those who, after a life of uprightness and rectitude, become, in middle age or later, perverted in conduct, and take to criminal and immoral practices, which, as in moral imbecility, punishment and exposure are ineffectual to arrest.
>
> (Mercier 1911: 250ff)

Mercier, physician in mental diseases at Charing Cross Hospital, here recognises medicine's interest in the phenomenon of imbecility and moral imbecility and its prior existence as a 'mental affection'.

But with the disaggregation of the asylum population, moral imbecility, as a continuum of imbecility, came increasingly to be construed as the object of 'training', rather than medical 'treatment'. The continuum of imbecility and moral imbecility was enshrined in the English *Report of the Royal Commission on the Care and Control of the Feeble-minded* (1908) and was used for the next two decades or more in both England and Australia as an authoritative set of classifications to underpin special education provision. In the 1929 *Report of Mental*

Deficiency in the Commonwealth of Australia (Ernest Jones 1929), for example, 'moral deficients' made up a fourth class of the feeble-minded much the same as in the 1908 English report. By this stage it was considered quite inappropriate that mental deficients should fall under the Lunacy Act or should share institutional arrangements with the mentally ill. Specific tools of measurement were taken up in order to deal, in educational terms, with a group whose administrative separation from medical institutions was already well under way. As it became possible through the development of these tools to identify the deficient and defective, it also became possible to know this group as distinct from the insane and to know them by means of techniques distinct from medicine. Such tools were to be provided by an emergent psychology, and in the name of education.

Medical science, of course, did not relinquish the field at all. On the contrary, psychology inherited from physiology a model for under-standing behaviour in the form of the reflex nervous system, and from statistics it gained a means of developing a more complex and relational conception of behaviour. Reflexology, the study of the reflex nervous system, provided the basic 'atom' or unit by which behaviour could begin to be counted. This included behaviour which was thought to be entirely independent of the brain or the will yet could still be measured, such as the classic 'knee-jerk reaction'. It also took in behaviour which might be seen to circumvent rational or prudent judgement. In Australia, R.J.A. Berry, professor of anatomy at Melbourne University, developed this model most fully. For him, grades of mental defectiveness could be constructed which corresponded to the network of neuronic arcs, and his hierarchical scale of idiot, imbecile and high-grade moron were directly proportional to the intricacy of the neuronic arcs – or pathways – involved from stimulus to response. Hence his belief that cranial capacity existed in direct proportion to mental capacity (Berry 1924: 393ff). According to Berry's schema, the high-grade moron, or moral imbecile, was the outcome of a physiological defect – a truncated pattern of neuronic pathways, which, though less gross than other grades of defectiveness, narrowed the gap between stimulus and response, that gap in which the 'moral' qualities of prudence, forethought and judgement could take place. Cleckley's version of psychopathic personality was an example of such reflexivity in the extreme; the psychopath was not a 'complete' man at all, but something resembling 'a subtly constructed reflex machine which can mimic the human personality perfectly' (Cleckley 1941: 398; Bleechmore 1975: 37–8).

The physiological model of units of human action, which makes possible a breakdown of responses into quantifiable, 'serialised' behaviour, lends many of the tools which allowed psychology to take off in its own direction (Danziger 1990: 139). 'Pure' physiology was interested in articulating behaviour in terms of stimulus and response and then measuring the gap between these two as a way of understanding the physical pathway that separated them. Psychology used that same articulation of stimulus and response but interpreted this in terms of what took place between them into 'experience' and later 'performance'. As a result, an individual gradually was able to be endowed with a particular 'capacity'. These transmutations allowed for the possibility of being deficient in capacity, and it was through the development of such tools that the 'mentally deficient' became known. The category of moral imbecility was a precursor to personality disorder but was calculated on a grid of the mentally deficient/ defective.

The movement of the defective out of the category of the insane was made possible by the use of tools for measuring intellectual capacity, such as those developed by Binet, who clearly saw himself at the educationists' disposal and having little to do with medicine. But there was by now clear evidence that the tool, as a linear gauge, proved too narrow for the requirements of researchers wanting to predict success at given tasks which depended on specific personal qualities rather than simply intellectual capacities. Danziger summed it up: an ability to solve quasi-scholastic problems with unambiguous right or wrong answers counted for little in deciding on leadership qualities or choosing an effective salesman. The initial work in the psy-disciplines, however, focused more on those groups which needed to be managed (Rose 1985, 1988, 1990). More 'space' was needed to incorporate a group previously but inadequately known as 'defective' or 'deficient' whose administration had early been recognised as a problem. That pioneer of educational measurement, Alfred Binet, observed in 1905 the limitations of the intellectual measure in attempting to define 'the present mental state' of the child:

> in the definition of this state, we should make some restrictions. Most subnormal children, especially those in schools, are habitually grouped in two categories, those of backward intelligence, and those who are unstable. This latter class, which certain alienists call moral imbeciles, do not necessarily manifest inferiority of intelligence: they are turbulent, vicious, rebellious to all discipline; they lack

sequence of ideas, and probably power of attention. . . . It would necessitate a long study, and probably a very difficult one, to establish the distinctive signs which separate the unstable from the undisciplined.

(Binet and Simon 1905: 37)

From the inception of the intelligence test, a group was recognised that, although generally conceived as sitting atop the hierarchy of mental defectiveness–deficiency, nevertheless sat in an uneasy relation to the overall category (McCallum 1990). Measurements of mental capacity, rather than leading to a thorough knowledge of this liminal group, tended to put a question-mark over its identifiability, progressively hewing it off from the main population of defectives–deficients. This group was unable to be known and governed using the existing technology applied to the overall classification.

Emerging from this separated group of defectives and deficients came the 'psychopathic personality', but it too comes to be understood with yet another set of tools, this time provided by the psychology of personality. This category of person emerged out of the category of the defective, as is clear from successive entries in the *Annual Reports* of the New South Wales Mental Hygiene Authority. The call in 1934, under the heading 'Mental Defectives Act', was for special legislation to deal effectively with mental defectives and for building institutions for mental defectives, in the name of the 'integrity of the mental and physical standard of the race' (New South Wales Mental Hygiene Authority, *Annual Report* 1934). In the following year, provision for criminal patients was deemed inadequate in that 'many persons who should have been dealt with in hospitals have been required to remain in gaols', and consequently a new hospital for criminals was opened at Morisset (New South Wales Mental Hygiene Authority, *Annual Report* 1935). The next year saw the arrival of a special institution at Morisset, with the emphasis on transferring mental defectives out of psychiatric institutions and providing them with educational services. The word 'control' is used repeatedly, not 'care' or 'treatment', indicating the shift of this category of persons outside of the medical framework of understanding. From 1937 until 1940 there were repetitions of earlier calls for adequate legislation and institutions to deal with the mental defective, but with a new emphasis on the 'control of higher-grade mental defectives' who were beyond the control of education or child welfare. There was also now mention of the Mental Defectives (Convicted Persons) Act 1939, still under the Lunacy Act but with the unequivocal recognition that this group is 'not insane' (New South Wales Mental Hygiene Authority, *Annual Report* 1940). By 1946, however, there was an attempt at clarifying and delimiting a group which to that point still defies definite classification:

> The definition of a 'mentally defective person' laid down by the [Mental Defective (Convicted Persons)] Act is somewhat narrow, implying only the criterion of inherent intellectual defect. The Act should be amended so as to embrace individuals neither mentally defective nor insane, but who come within the category of psychopathic personalities.
>
> (New South Wales Mental Hygiene Authority,
> *Annual Report* 1946)

The space turned to, in a way which extended the use of a particular language and conceptual terrain allowing for the calculation of all individuals, was that of personality. Personality sought to grasp that which failed to be captured in the more defined categories of insanity or defectiveness, but also that which could be measured in the ranks of the normal, across the whole population. Danziger's work on the history of psychological research is useful in showing the transformation from a single dimension of performance, as represented in the intelligence test, to a more complex register of human capacities with multiple lines to gauge multiple performances. The space which became personality was in fact the outcome of historically specific techniques of calculation and marking out spaces (Armstrong 1993).

CONCLUSION

Much of the existing certainty and truthfulness of the category of personality and personality disorder is disturbed by attempts to map out a genealogical analysis of its contemporary uses. Rather than the natural, ahistorical contents of one's individuality, the category of personality is understood here as the result of certain historical contingencies; first, the increased individualisation of the population accomplished in the late nineteenth century through statistical procedures and administrative reforms such as schooling, health and other social hygiene strategies designed to map the interstices between people (Hacking 1990; Armstrong 1993); second, the production of knowledge concerned with the internal dimensions of individuality in all its complexity, which is associated with the growth of the psy-disciplines during the twentieth century (Rose 1985, 1990; McCallum

1990); and third, the late twentieth-century objectives of political power to regulate citizens through the advancement of norms of personal life, such as the forging of a desire towards the shaping and presentation of a well-adjusted personality.

The historical approach outlined in this chapter attempts to show how the conceptual terrain for thinking and acting upon the problem of the dangerous individual is the product of governmental attempts to know and understand persons. It suggests that knowledge of particular types of persons is made possible by means of a complexity of interrelations between law and psychiatry and the institutional spaces in which they operate, rather than the happenstance discoveries of the human sciences or essential properties of persons described in law or medicine. This 'psychiatrization of criminal danger' (Foucault 1988: 128) involved a collaboration over new techniques of management focusing on the instincts, motivations and will of individuals needing to be transformed.

ACKNOWLEDGEMENTS

My thanks to Jennifer Laurence for her assistance with this work, and to the Australian Research Council for its support for this project.

REFERENCES

American Psychiatric Association (1982) *Diagnostic and Statistical Manual of Mental Disorders (3rd edition revised)*, Washington DC: American Psychiatric Association.

Armstrong, D. (1993) 'Public health spaces and the fabrication of identity', *Sociology*, 27, 3: 393–410.

Bartholomew, A. and Milte, K. (1976) 'The reliability and validity of psychiatric diagnoses in courts of law', *The Australian Law Journal*, 50: 450–8.

Berry, R.J.A. (1924) 'The correlation of recent advances in cerebral structure and function with feeble-mindedness and its diagnostic applicability', *Medical Journal of Australia*, 7 June: 393ff.

Binet, A. and Simon, T. (1905) 'New methods for the diagnosis of the intellectual level of sub-normals', in *The Development of Intelligence in Children*, New Jersey: Vineland Training School.

Blackstone, W. (1972) *Commentaries on the Laws of England, 1765–9*, Oxford: Oxford University Press.

Bleechmore, J.F. (1975) 'Towards a rational theory of criminal responsibility: the psychopathic offender', *Melbourne University Law Review*, 10, 1: 19–46.

Bostock, J. (1968) *The Dawn of Australian Psychiatry*, Sydney: Medical Publishing Company.

Burchell, G. (1993) 'Liberal government and techniques of the self', *Economy and Society*, 22, 3: 267–82.

Campbell, I.G. (1988) *Mental Disorder and Criminal Law in Australia and New Zealand*, Sydney: Butterworths.

Cleckley, H. (1941) *The Mask of Sanity: An Attempt to Clarify Some Issues about the So-called Psychopathic Personality*, St Louis: C.V. Mosby and Co.

Cocozza, J. and Steadman, H. (1976) 'The failure of psychiatric predictions of dangerousness: clear and convincing evidence', *Rutgers Law Review*, 30: 1084–101.

Coppe, L. (1986) 'Insane or greatly injured? The Captain Hyndman case', in 1838 volume, Collective of Australian Bicentennial History, *The Push from the Bush*, 23: 55–7.

Cummins, C.J. (1967) *The Administration of Lunacy and Idiocy in New South Wales 1788–1855*, Sydney: NSW Department of Public Health.

Danziger, K. (1990) *Constructing the Subject. Historical Origins of Psychological Research*, New York: Cambridge University Press.

Dax, E. Cunningham (1981) 'Crimes, follies and misfortunes in the history of Australasian psychiatry', *Australian and New Zealand Journal of Psychiatry*, 15: 257–63.

Deleuze, G. (1993) *Foucault*, Minnesota: University of Minnesota Press.

Ellard, J. (1989) *Some Rules for Killing People*, Sydney: Angus and Robertson.

Ellis, A.S. (1983) *Eloquent Testimony: The Story of the Mental Health Services in Western Australia*, Nedlands: University of Western Australia Press.

Ernest Jones, W. (1929) *Report of Mental Deficiency in the Commonwealth of Australia*, Canberra: H.J. Green Government Printer.

Fairall, P. (1993) 'Violent offenders and community protection in Victoria – the Gary David experience', *Criminal Law Journal*, 17: 40–54.

Floud, J. and Young, W. (1981) *Dangerousness and Criminal Justice*, Heinemann: London.

Foucault, M. (1965) *Madness and Civilization*, trans. R. Howard, New York: Vintage.

Foucault, M. (1980) 'Body/power', in C. Gordon (ed.) *Power/Knowledge: Selected Interviews and Other Writings by Michel Foucault, 1972–1977*, New York: Pantheon.

Foucault, M. (1988) 'The dangerous individual', in L.D. Kritzman (ed.) *Michel Foucault: Politics, Philosophy, Culture*, New York: Routledge.

Foucault, M. (1991) 'Questions of method', in G. Burchell, C. Gordon and P. Miller (eds) *The Foucault Effect: Studies in Governmentality*, London: Harvester Wheatsheaf.

Garton, S. (1982) '"Bad or mad". Developments in incarceration in NSW', in Sydney Labour History Group *What Rough Beast? The State and Social Order in Australian History*, Sydney: Allen and Unwin.

Glaser, W. (1990) 'Morality and medicine', *Legal Service Bulletin*, 15, 3: 114–16.

Glaser, W. (1994) 'Commentary: Gary David, psychiatry, and the discourse of dangerousness', *Australian and New Zealand Journal of Criminology*, 27: 46–9.

Gordon, C. (1990) '*Histoire de la folie*: an unknown book by Michel Foucault', *History of the Human Sciences*, 3, 1: 3–26.

Gutting, G. (1994) 'Foucault and the history of madness', in G. Gutting (ed.)

The Cambridge Companion to Foucault, Cambridge: Cambridge University Press.

Hacking, I. (1986) 'Making up people', in T. Heller, S. Morton and D. Wellber (eds) *Reconstructing Individualism: Autonomy, Individuality and the Self in Western Thought*, Stanford: Stanford University Press.

Hacking, I. (1990) *The Taming of Chance*, Cambridge: Cambridge University Press.

Historical Records of Australia (1914) Series 1, Governors' Despatches to and from England, vol. 1, 1788–1796, The Library Committee of the Commonwealth Parliament, 2–8.

Kissane, K. (1990) 'Are they mad or bad? Lawyers and psychiatrists differ on how to protect society from violent psychopaths', *Time Australia*, 135, 5 (June): 42–3.

Law Reform Commission of Victoria (1990) *The Concept of Mental Illness in the 'Mental Health Act' 1980*, Report No. 31, Melbourne: Government Printer.

McCallum, D. (1990) *The Social Production of Merit. Education, Psychology and Politics in Australia, 1900–1950*, London: Falmer.

Mercier, C. (1911) *Crime and Insanity*, London: Williams and Norgate.

Midelfort, H.C. Eric (1980) 'Madness and civilisation in early modern Europe: a reappraisal of Michel Foucault', in B. Malament (ed.) *After the Reformation: Essays in Honor of J.H. Hexter*, Philadelphia: University of Philadelphia Press.

Miller, P. and Rose, N. (1988) 'The Tavistock Program: the government of subjectivity and social life', *Sociology*, 22, 2: 171–92.

Miller, P. and Rose, N. (1990) 'Governing economic life', *Economy and Society*, 19, 1: 1–31.

Minson, J. (1985) *Genealogies of Morals. Nietzsche, Foucault, Donzelot and the Eccentricity of Ethics*, New York: St Martin's Press.

New South Wales Mental Hygiene Authority, *Annual Reports*, 1934–1950, Sydney: Government Printer.

O'Brien, P. (1989) 'Michel Foucault's history of culture', in Lynn Hunt (ed.) *The New Cultural History*, Berkeley: University of California Press.

O'Sullivan, J. (1981) *Mental Health and the Law*, Sydney: The Law Book Company.

Parker, N. (1991) 'The Gary David case', *Australian and New Zealand Journal of Psychiatry*, 25: 371–4.

Reid, W. (1985) 'Psychopathy and dangerousness', in M. Roth and R. Blugrass (eds) *Psychiatry, Human Rights and the Law*, Cambridge: Cambridge University Press.

Report of the Royal Commission on the Care and Control of the Feeble-minded (1908) London: HMSO.

Rose, N. (1985) *The Psychological Complex: Psychology, Politics and Society in England, 1869–1939*, London: Routledge and Kegan Paul.

Rose, N. (1988) 'Calculable minds and manageable individuals', *History of the Human Sciences*, 1: 179–200.

Rose, N. (1990) *Governing the Soul: The Shaping of the Private Self*, London: Routledge.

Victoria, Inspector-General of Insane, *Annual Reports*, 1905–1933.

Weeks, J. (1982) 'Foucault for historians', *History Workshop*, 14: 106–19.
Williams, C. R. (1990) 'Psychopathy, mental illness and preventive detention: issues arising from the David case', *Monash University Law Review*, 16, 2: 161–83.

Chapter 4

At risk of maladjustment
The problem of child mental health

Deborah Tyler

A Melbourne mother resting in hospital after the birth of her son was brought a screaming infant (Heath 1995: 4). Without looking at the child, she told the nurse the baby was not hers, and asked her to take the baby away. An alarming tale of post-natal depression, or of the failure of a mother to bond with her new-born? Not at all. The mother, Glenis Dolphin, simply knew that the child was not hers. Her baby was 'placid and easy-going' and 'did not cry'.

Ten years down the track, her child, Sam, is still easy-going. Lucky Sam is blessed with a temperament, an 'overall behavioural style' (Sanson *et al.* 1990: 181) that means that a cheery, stable and successful adult life is taken to be a relatively assured outcome. And he is also blessed with a mother as knowledgeable about her child and child development as Glenis Dolphin; a mother who, when confronted with a crying baby, knew this was not her son, was not perturbed by a 10-year-old's friendships with older men, and who has not sought to produce an intense 'mother–son' relationship. A mother who knew that the physical manifestation of headaches was a sign of emotional distress, indicating a lack of fit between Sam and his school. A mother who acted promptly and without fuss and found him a more suitable environment.

This tale of the good mother and the perfect child comes to us courtesy of the Australian Temperament Project (ATP) (Prior 1989, 1992). Sam, along with 2,500 other Victorian children born in the mid-1980s, is having his path from babyhood through childhood monitored in an investigation funded through the National Health and Medical Research Council. The project began with the premise that each person is the bearer of a particular temperament, an in-born tendency to respond to events and experiences in consistent, stable and predictable ways. It aims to monitor the bearers of different habitual styles of behaviour in their engagements with the tasks of growing up. While the

ATP has found that some temperaments are naturally more advantageous than others – to be sociable is preferable to being withdrawn – the larger issue determining the path through childhood is the 'degree of fit' between temperament and environment, including the human environment.

Perhaps the most surprising 'discovery' of the research so far, and certainly that which has received most publicity, is the identification of boys as a problem population, significantly less competent at managing the developmental challenges of childhood than girls (Heath 1995; Legge 1995; Sanson *et al.* 1993; Sweet 1995). In statistical terms, the profile of the competent child – flexible, adaptable, sociable, self-regulating, who can expect to 'flourish throughout life' – is more likely to belong to Samantha than Sam. By the age of 12, boys are twice as likely as girls to have behaviour problems. Boys who make trouble turn out to be troubled boys, or as one Australian national daily put it 'Boys: sadder and badder than girls' (Sweet 1995). While studies of children identified clinically as having behavioural and learning problems have consistently noted that boys are in the majority, the specific contribution of the ATP has been to pinpoint the development of gender disparities in the behavioural styles of the non-clinical population of 'normal children' through a longitudinal study. To employ a well-worn metaphor, those boys whose difficulties are severe enough to come to the attention of specialists are merely the visible tip of a much larger iceberg, and of a much larger problem. Troubled boys can be expected to grow into troublesome men.

Connections have been made between the statistical picture of sad and bad little boys produced by the ATP, and the findings of other investigations: the higher suicide rates of young males, the greater presence of males in prisons (and detention classes), and the disproportionate involvement of males in forms of conduct which violate a range of social norms:

> By adulthood, males are responsible for almost all violent crimes, and for a variety of other aggressive behaviours such as domestic violence, child abuse, drink driving, and road accidents.
>
> (Sanson *et al.* 1993: 86)

For parents the message is clear. The project leader Professor Margot Prior 'urged parents of "difficult-to-manage toddlers" to get help early because early intervention paid big dividends'. And:

> Parents wanting to do the best for their children need only do one

thing – treat them like young girls whatever their sex. Ask them to be responsible, caring and nurturing. Expect them to be sharing and able to manage themselves.

(Heath 1995: 4)

While treating boys like girls might appear to be a risky business to many Australian parents, according to the ATP the risks to future well-being engendered by treating boys like boys are more firmly grounded. Perhaps one of the peculiarities of the present is that this advice is both intelligible and potentially able to be acted upon. But a further peculiarity is that, only a decade ago, parents wanting to do the best for their daughters were urged to treat them like young boys.

At first glance, the designation of girls as 'better children' than boys appears to be a radical overturning of much of the recent past. Indeed, Valerie Walkerdine, in a valuable analysis appearing in the mid-1980s, concluded that in developmental terms the likelihood of performing successfully as both a 'child' and as a 'girl' was remote (Walkerdine 1985). Walkerdine demonstrated that modern conceptions of child development take children to be by nature active, enquiring and heading steadily towards autonomy as an adult. But the behaviours associated with being a good 'girl', heading steadily towards a nurturing competence and desired styles of adult femininity, she argued, are at odds with the characteristics of the 'child'. According to Walkerdine, girls are located educationally at the intersection of two competing discourses, a location where 'their position as children must remain shaky and partial, continually played across by their position as feminine' (Walkerdine 1985: 210). But there is no doubt that, according to the findings of the ATP, girls are 'better children' than boys. Further, those same attributes that Walkerdine identifies as excluding girls from the ranks of competent children are precisely those cited by the ATP as the hallmarks of the competent child.

Clearly, the disjuncture between Walkerdine's analysis of the positioning of girls as less competent at the work of being a child and the ATP's 'discovery' that it is boys who are less competent requires explanation. The ATP's disconcerting admission that 'we cannot specify what it [temperament] is' (Prior 1992: 95), alongside its claims to an expanded territory ranging from screaming babies to drunk drivers and violent men where the expertise of psychologists might profitably be employed, might make the ATP appear an apt target for the kind of socio-cultural critique generally directed at the psychological sciences (Rose 1988), even without the sense of perturbation created by its 'discovery' of boys as a problem population. Yet, I suggest accounts framed by the traditions of socio-cultural critique are limited in their usefulness for understanding either the contemporary significance of the ATP, the recent past of developmental and child psychology, or the field of mental health.

An alternative starting point is to take seriously the possibility that girls and boys might indeed exchange positions as problem populations within the space of a decade. The task of this chapter is to utilise historical investigations to explain, rather than explain away, this possibility. Such an approach involves unsettling the claims of the ATP to be enquiring further into a little-understood zone of the human mind, to be learning more about 'temperament' or, for that matter, about inner secrets which make boys and girls tick in different ways. But the ATP, I suggest, ought be taken less as an exemplary instance of child psychology's wrong-headedness than an exemplary contemporary example of the imbrication of child psychology in the arts of modern government.

We operate in a present where, in the psychological domain, being a child has been produced as a restricted competence, a present where some children are better at being children than others, and where it is possible to calculate success or failure at the work of being a child. We operate in a present where it is possible to conceptualise children as the bearers of 'an overall behavioural style' and where the troubles of children and adults alike are made intelligible through the single plane of 'maladjustment'. This chapter seeks to lay bare the formation of these contours of the present by investigating how questions of conduct have come to be posed in these ways. The sense of perturbation produced by the ATP's problematisation of male conduct and its casting of boys as a population at risk of maladjustment provides an opportunity to reconsider the usefulness of taking the existence of sexually differentiated populations as fixed points in determining the shape of those contours. To borrow from Denise Riley, it may be possible to catch more than once the category of girls 'on the wings of its formation' as a distinct population with specifiable attributes (Riley 1988: 103). The same may be the case for boys.

Michel Foucault suggested that his work ought be taken not as a set of 'dogmatic assertions' but as 'openings . . . where those who may be interested are invited to join in' (Foucault 1981: 4). Before joining in, then, I want to indicate those aspects of Foucault's thinking that I have taken as openings to mount an enquiry into child psychology and into the production of gendered populations in directions foreclosed by socio-cultural critique.

HISTORIES OF THE PRESENT

Foucault advocated the utilisation of historical investigations as a tool for 'diagnosing the present' (Foucault 1977). For Foucault, the task of historical investigations lies in making the contours of the present strange, rather than the past familiar. For this task, the demand that the work of the historian lies in uncovering a substratum of sameness that leads inexorably to the present must be put to one side. Historical investigations, when chance and contingency are given their due, may be mobilised to the work of unsettling – rather than bolstering – current certainties. Histories of the present, as work conducted in this vein have come to be known, work to disturb the taken-for-grantedness and self-evidence of the present, work, in Foucault's words to 'show that things "weren't as necessary as all that"' (Foucault 1981: 12). In the context of the contemporary problems whose outlines I have sketched above, then, Foucault's approach to the making of histories offers an invitation to disturb the naturalness and self-evident character of 'the child', 'boys' and 'girls' as pre-given objects of study, as always existing objects about whom child psychology produces more or less adequate accounts. Unsettling the stability of child psychology's objects of study assists in making visible the processes through which psychology produces the objects about which it speaks. And it is here that a further strand of Foucault's work, the arena of enquiry that he neologised as 'governmentality', has a part to play.

Foucault offered a set of related formulations to describe 'governmentality'. In 'On governmentality' the term is employed to describe the eighteenth-century emergence of an art of government organised around the maximisation of the capacities of populations, and to draw attention to those techniques which have made it possible for populations to enter into the calculations of political rule (Foucault 1976). Nikolas Rose has added to this a reminder of the modern statistical formulation of population as a 'bounded field', whose characteristics can be grasped through the concept of the norm, with a regular distribution of variations. Population as a bounded field makes it possible to understand the existence of particular populations with differing characteristics, subject to different regulatory practices aimed at a range of outcomes (Rose 1985: 64–5). Populations exist, for example, within schools or as a target of policy, as well as within national boundaries.

For populations to become an object of political thought and intervention requires knowledge of the field to be acted upon. Thus the work of modern government is literally and figuratively unthinkable without the techniques of statistics, techniques through which the characteristics of the population are inscribed in a numerical form. We need only note the extent to which investigations like the ATP are massive data collection exercises, recording the emotional and behavioural attributes of children, to establish one frame through which the psychological sciences are bound up in programmes of government. There is nothing inherently 'psychological' about these techniques: they become 'psychological' only at the moment of their application to the inner, emotional life of future citizens. We might also note the routine appearance of 'the child' of child psychology within institutional settings, and equally the routine application of psychological expertise to the problems of managing particular child populations.

But the ambitions of political authorities are not achieved through a mere registration of the presence or absence of desired attributes amongst target populations. The rationale of government is to maximise the capacities of populations: an art of facilitating the development of certain characteristics, and of eliminating or minimising the presence of others. In one of his later formulations, Foucault defined govern-mentality as the 'contact' between technologies of power which 'determine the conduct of individuals and submit them to certain ends or domination' and technologies of the self:

> which permit individuals to effect by their own means or with the help of others a certain number of operations on their own bodies and souls, thoughts, conduct and way of being, so as to transform themselves in order to attain a certain state of happiness, wisdom, perfection, or immortality.
>
> (Foucault 1988: 18)

Or, one might add, the achievement of a degree of 'fit' between oneself and one's environment. On one level it is of course pure serendipity that Foucault's conception of a 'contact' between technologies of domination and technologies of the self is echoed quite so strongly in the ATP's work of calibration of levels of self-regulation amongst sexually differentiated child populations, and its registration of the existence of problem behaviour through care-givers' ratings of ease of management, teacher's assessments of the capacity to 'adapt to the demands of the classroom' and so on. Or is it? On another level, this echoing suggests a second frame through which child psychology might be imbricated in the arts of government. The terrain of child psychology may be understood as, on the one hand, a set of techniques for registering the distribution of valued and unwanted attributes across child populations. And, on the other, it may be understood as a certain kind of expertise, a practical know-how which acts to shape the conduct of others through providing guidance on how to fashion the self-conduct of children in desired directions.

Foucault's work presents ample openings for thinking about the ATP and about how, in the space of a decade, girls and boys might exchange positions as problem populations. But we have gone as far as we ought in advance of historical investigation of the formation of present certainties. Let me turn now to the recent past, and in particular to those settings where it has been found helpful to conceptualise children as the bearers of an overall behavioural style, to the conditions which have made it possible to do so, and to the development of techniques through which that style might be realigned.

THE HISTORY OF A PERSONALITY

In 1935, Professor W.S. Dawson opened a discussion on the 'Psychoses of adolescence' at the British Medical Association (Australian Division) Annual Conference. Dawson argued that the way forward in understanding both dementia praecox and manic depression lay in the study of the personality before the onset of psychoses:

> Many patients displayed a fundamental lack of adaptability and from early years had seemed incapable of competing on equal terms with their fellows. The history of a personality which was inadequate in the emotional rather than in the purely intellectual field was sufficiently common to be significant. . . . From a preventive point of view, it would appear that the recognition of these types in early childhood and the correction of anomalies in character was of supreme importance.
>
> (Dawson 1935: 479)

Dr C. Farran-Ridge (1935: 479) suggested that the 'pre-disposed' should be taught 'boxing and ju-jitsu, elocution and public speaking' to combat their 'natural timidity'. Other doctors were more alert to the nature of the problem of prevention that Dawson posed: the need for development of techniques by which the 'pre-disposed' could be recognised before their 'anomalies' became too habitual; the development of corrective strategies through which the 'history of a personality' would be written differently. Training the timid youth in ju-jitsu and boxing was too little and too late.

How then might the ordinary doctor, or the psychiatrist, come to recognise the 'pre-disposed', when the task of making accurate diagnoses of adolescents actually manifesting psychotic behaviour was so difficult? How would the doctor even come into contact with the 'pre-disposed' before the onset of illness? Dr A.W. Campbell put the problem clearly when he asked:

> whether personality traits observed in children could enable one to foretell the onset of dementia praecox. His experience at the Royal Alexandra Hospital for Children in Sydney had not enabled him to say that he could. He realised that the wards of children's hospitals were not the right places for obtaining the necessary data. Nor could one rely on the memory of parents. The desire of a child to escape from the paternal presence was no indication of a psychosis.
>
> (Campbell 1935: 479)

Campbell's comment that hospital wards were not the 'right places' for observing the occurrence of personality traits from which the future might be predicted is worth attending to. Such settings were too far removed from the child's normal environment, and were threatening in ways that made fearfulness, timidity, sleep disturbances, bed-wetting and so on likely responses of children who might not display such behaviours outside the hospital. Further, the kind of data routinely assembled by medical personnel on the physically ill child was of the wrong sort, concerned only with observations bearing on the child's physical welfare and covering only the time-span of hospitalisation.

Three years after Dawson had introduced the problem, John Williams, psychiatrist at the Children's Hospital in Melbourne, expressed his concern that the medical profession was missing out on opportunities to do important work in the recognition, prevention and treatment of behavioural problems (Williams 1938: 145–8). Once again, medical environments were the wrong place to be because 'the hurried atmosphere of the consulting room' did not provide a space where the child could be observed over time, nor a setting where habitual behaviours might be forthcoming, nor one free of 'the inhibiting effect of the presence of parents'. But the most intransigent problem, Williams argued, was the simple ignorance of doctors of the field of child development, coupled with 'an inability to visualise the child as anything but a collection of organs which each may become diseased and require treatment'. The medical profession must 'fit itself for the treatment of such problems' or others would take the lead.

Others of course had already taken the lead. As early as 1932 K.S.

Cunningham, in his report on 'Problem children in Melbourne schools' prepared for the Victorian Council of Mental Hygiene, had been able to report on the numbers of pre-school children displaying the kind of behaviour traits that Dawson had suggested were precursors of serious mental instability in adolescence (Cunningham 1932: 75–85). Cunningham's report was an investigation of the need for the establishment of child guidance clinics in Melbourne, and calculated the incidence of problems that such a clinic could be expected to address occurring in all types of schools, covering all age ranges. His data on 'conduct disorders', including truancy, temper, bullying, deceitfulness and sulkiness, drew on teachers' returns from the spectrum of existing institutions; charitable institutions, kindergartens, technical schools, state schools and private schools. For his data on 'habits', including nightmares and nervous habits, and personality defects where the categories ran to the neurotic, hyperactive, hypokinetic, seclusive, egocentric, inadequate and cyclothymic he was able to draw only on returns from kindergartens and children's institutions.

Kindergarten teachers in 1932 were not themselves classifying the children they observed into the categories utilised by Cunningham. The clusters were his own with the definitions supplied to the teacher. So a child would be classified as 'emotional' if he or she 'laughs and cries too easily, [was] readily excited and upset, over-sensitive, easily discouraged', as 'seclusive' if he/she 'plays alone, day-dreams, [was] shy, quiet or reserved' (Cunningham 1932: 78). Each category was made up of a number of sub-sections, and to be constituted as a 'problem child' required the habitual display of more than one 'abnormality'. But, though Cunningham provided the categories, kindergarten teachers were by 1932 able to visualise children as the bearers of an overall behavioural style.

For Cunningham, the survey left no doubt that Melbourne required child guidance clinics under the auspices of the Victorian Council for Mental Hygiene. Our interest in his survey is a little different. First, while the problem of how to recognise the 'pre-disposed' was one that eluded the combined talents of the Australian medical profession, Melbourne kindergarten teachers were, without apparent difficulty, recognising and classifying children according to various behaviours understood to lead to adult inefficiencies. The kindergarten teacher was able to 'visualise' the child in ways that the medical profession could not; under her gaze hitherto hidden features of the child were made visible. Second, her powers of observation exceeded those of the teacher of older children operating in the milieu of the state school. The state school teacher was able to observe only 'bad conduct' where the boundaries of 'good behaviour' were crossed. The kindergarten teacher was able to supply, in addition, data on defects of personality and habit, which attended to the way that the child met the challenges of the kindergarten environment. Third, the kindergarten population was composed of 'normal' children, or at least comprised only those children whose intellectual capacity was judged as able to meet the demands of a normal environment. The explanation for the 'lack of fit' displayed by some children to the kindergarten environment was not supplied by intelligence tests, which were still, in the early 1930s, synonymous with 'psychology'. Fourth, the kindergarten was understood not only to provide the setting which made visible behaviour problems in young children, but also to offer a milieu for the reshaping of conduct in more desired directions.

THE KINDERGARTEN

How had kindergartens become the 'right places' for those concerned with the conduct of young children to be? Let us follow the lead provided by child psychiatrists and educational psychologists and turn our attention, albeit briefly, to the inter-war kindergartens and nursery schools.

Kindergartens and nursery schools had been a recognised tool of social reform in Australia since the late nineteenth century. Early kindergartens were a philanthropic response to the newly visible conditions of 'slum' childhoods. In the early decades of the twentieth century, the kindergarten worker was able to understand herself as having a beneficial effect through her missionary activities in the child's home, and through the exercise of her capacities to make an alternative home with herself at its centre. As a figure of emulation, the success of her efforts was measured by the knowledge that she stayed in the child's mind as a vision of what could be. But by the mid-1920s any teacher who sought to place herself at the centre of the child's day was failing her profession.

Elements of the transformation of the kindergarten worker from a figure of emulation to an observer of children are provided by Mary Lush's *Progressive Kindergarten Methods*, a training manual published in 1926. Lush provided a series of questions for the worker to reflect upon her practice so that she might become 'an artist in her profession'. Her first question, 'Is my attitude to the children, "Let us find out what this creature does?" Or do I "teach" the children?', not only invited those who thought of their work in terms of teaching to think again, but established the proper way of thinking about kindergarten children (Lush 1926: 26). They were to be approached as unfamiliar beings, as 'creatures' to be observed and studied in order that nature and habits could be made known. While there were many ways in which a kindergarten worker could fail, '[t]he one teacher who above all others is a failure is the teacher who knows it all' (Lush 1926: 158).

While the transformation of the kindergarten worker from a teacher to an observer of children was central to the possibility of conceptualising children as the bearers of an overall behavioural style, it would be a mistake to assume that such outcomes were intended. The relationship I am describing is not one of cause and effect, but one of unplanned and unforeseeable outcomes. The impetus shaping the reformation of the kindergarten was merely to make more effective its work of shaping the conduct of children in ways that could be expected to carry over into the conduct of adult life.

Lush herself, in the mid-1920s, was quite clear in her assessment of the limits of psychology's existing tools for assisting the worker in her task of 'learning to know the children better' (Lush 1926: 29). In 1917 she had visited the 'kindergarten laboratories' attached to Yale and Columbia Universities, where developmental psychology found its object of study (Rose 1989: 142–50). Developmental psychology had by the mid-1920s begun to establish age-related norms of activities to be mastered, and was of immediate practical value in constructing an environment where 'children really have an opportunity to pass from a lower to a higher stage' (Lush 1926: 9). 'Mental tests' had their uses but:

> these tests are not wholly satisfactory, because they exaggerate the importance of the purely intellectual equipment of the child, and do not take account of the total individuality.

> (Lush 1926: 147)

The limitations of mental tests for kindergarten work were not something that 'psychology' could be looked to for a remedy. In any case, other techniques – skilled observation of the child at play, alone and with others – were available to make known the 'non-intellectual equipment'. These techniques have now of course become part of the stock-in-trade of child psychologists. But they were not invented in the laboratory, nor were they privileged by Lush in any way as 'psychological'. Rather, such techniques formed part of the necessary 'equipment' of the kindergarten teacher, and were to be developed through her performance of certain kinds of work on the self.

The direction signalled by Lush's advice that workers should 'form the habit of systematically observing children' (1926: 169) before intervening was consolidated by the re-appointment of May Gutteridge as Principal of the Kindergarten Training College (KTC). Like Lush, Gutteridge had a long involvement with Melbourne kindergartens, and like Lush, she too had direct exposure to the American 'kindergarten laboratories', spending 1928–9 retraining at Columbia. On her return she established the newly purpose-built nursery school in inner-city Collingwood as a demonstration centre (Tyler 1993).

The new unit took children between 18 months and 3 years as its population, children for whom kindergarten training might otherwise come 'too late'. The centre aimed:

> to further the happy, harmonious development of *each* child in its care; to watch and study him, first, in order to progressively discover his individual needs, and then to provide him with opportunities to bring about a natural growth of body and mind.
>
> (Gutteridge 1932: 103)

These non-coercive techniques – observation, assessment, intervention – for the formation of desired attributes and the elimination of others in the conduct repertoire of individuals are familiar enough. The novelty of the work at Collingwood, in the Australian context, can be found less in the techniques utilised than in the age of the population to whom they were directed. The population was broken down further into separate groups of those from 18 to 24 months, 24–30 months and 30–36 months 'so that their development at each stage might be watched'. Staff were required to keep detailed records to give 'an exact picture of the child's actions as an expression of his development'. 'Development' not only included the growth of physical and intellectual prowess, but covered 'social' and 'emotional' development, with examples given of the kinds of behaviour to be recorded under each heading. Parents, too, were required to make 'simple home records', to provide the staff with 'records of sleep, elimination, food, as well as of emotional disturbances, such as temper, fear and of likes and dislikes'. Gutteridge's claims that 'the bond between the two [nursery school and home] has been strengthened in every possible way' and that the nursery school reached the child 'during the whole of his 24-hour day' were far from empty.

The nursery school had by the early 1930s commenced the kind of labour required to produce norms of emotional and social 'development'. By clustering children into age groups, providing an environment that constantly 'tested' the child and allowed success or failure to be observed, and recording the behaviours elicited, the child's conduct over time and space was able to be written down and made visible as an overall behavioural style and as a new narrative of development. Each child at the Collingwood Centre, from 18 months onwards, was the bearer of a personalised history of social and emotional adjustment, as well as of a history of physical and intellectual development. Those histories would accompany them from the nursery school into the kindergarten, and, potentially at least, travel further. A beginning had been made on establishing the 'history of a personality' that Dawson had suggested would assist in the management of troubled adolescents. Gutteridge advised that the records would be kept on file 'and can be further investigated by any who are interested in following the history of any child' (Gutteridge 1932: 109).

If recognition of certain 'types' of conduct in young children provided one half of Dawson's preventive equation, the correction of character 'anomalies' as soon as they became evident provided the other. The published records of individual children demonstrated how problem behaviours were able to be eliminated or at least minimised in frequency by 'adjusting' an individual child's environment, including the human environment. Negative children had been transformed in a few short months into children whose 'adjustment to other children and to adults is above average' (Gutteridge 1932: 113–24). The child whose problems proved too intractable, or whose constellation of negative attributes made the definition of the ground to be worked upon too opaque, would require further observation and more specialised assistance.

THE CHILDREN'S HOSPITAL PSYCHIATRIC CLINIC

By the early 1930s, John Williams, the Melbourne Children's Hospital psychiatrist who, as we have already heard, advised the medical profession to act quickly if they were to secure a new arena of activity, had himself already acted. His first task was to shift the pattern of referrals to the psychiatric clinic away from requests for assessments of suspected mentally deficient children, towards the assessment and treatment of children displaying behaviour problems (Williams 1932).

In 1932 Williams reported on the first 142 cases seen at the revamped Children's Hospital Psychiatric Clinic (Williams 1932: 294–9). In addition to Williams, the staff consisted of two psychologists and a social worker. The role of the psychologists was confined to 'mental tests of intelligence' with Williams assessing 'emotional difficulties'. The largest category of cases were those who were 'difficult to manage', classified by Williams as 'behaviour disorders'. He noted however that 'the demarcation between disorders of personality, behaviour and habit is not clear cut and is adopted for the sake of convenience'. Children did not fall readily under one or other heading, tending to display problems crossing the categories. Williams's table was, like Cunningham's, more a record of the presence of certain problems in a particular population, rather than a diagnosis of the individual. But while Williams had succeeded in taking the weight of clinical work away from the assessment of levels of mental deficiency, he conceded a certain amount of hopelessness about dealing effectively with the new population of 'behaviour problems':

> We often feel at the end of a long afternoon in the clinic that the parents are much more to blame than the children; and such complaints as 'difficult to manage', 'tantrums', and 'screaming fits' and so forth, often bring forth a history of a home environment in which even the most stable child would have a difficult task to make a satisfactory adaptation.
>
> (Williams 1932: 298)

Further, the child did not readily yield the secrets of its conduct to the clinical gaze, for, as Williams oberved:

> evaluation is extremely difficult. The obscurities of the motivation of conduct, the complexities of the child's mind, and the difficulties of approach may make the reconstruction of behaviour a task of great difficulty, requiring an even more delicate technique than that necessary with the adult.
>
> (Williams 1932: 299)

In 1932 all Williams's effort was directed towards trying to uncover the hidden 'why' of each individual child's behaviour, to reveal the inner secrets that made the child behave in a certain way. Finding 'why' would permit an accurate diagnosis to be made, from which an appropriate course of treatment could be expected to follow.

But by 1935, Williams was able to report on the outcomes on a new innovation in the techniques of clinical assessment and treatment of children with behaviour problems: the establishment of a nursery school within the psychiatric clinic. The nursery school differed from those outside the medical domain only in the selection of its population from those already assessed as requiring expert attention (Williams 1935).

The milieu of the nursery school/kindergarten proved to be readily transportable to the modern hospital. The quest for diagnostic accuracy preceded by the establishment of 'why' was no longer a preoccupation. It was, after all, not necessary to know the inner secrets of why children behaved as they did to be able to observe behavioural styles and to work on eliminating problem behaviours from the individual's repertoire. Williams advised Dawson, Campbell and others attending the forum on adolescent psychoses that he had indeed hoped that the nursery school would provide the appropriate conditions for 'observing abnormal personality traits' and establishing the history of a personality before the onset of psychotic behaviour. In the event, it had done much more:

> under the influence of nursery school conditions in which interference by adults was at a minimum, personality defects had become quickly modified, even those . . . who were probably pre-psychotic had recovered. Nursery schools were very important for the management of difficult children.
>
> (Williams 1935: 480)

Rather than simply providing the introduction to the history of a personality whose outlines could be predicted in advance, the nursery school offered the possibility of reshaping conduct, so that an apparently inevitable outcome need never occur. Treatment was possible and effective, and personalities could be reconstructed without ever precisely identifying the causation of the original fault-line.

Whereas in 1932 Williams had been confronted by 142 puzzling individuals who did not readily yield the secrets of their mental functioning, nor fall neatly into classifications, by the late 1930s all were made intelligible as demonstrating the same overall problem of maladjustment. In his 1938 report on the work undertaken at the Children's Hospital, Williams still spoke of children manifesting 'emotional difficulties', 'behaviour problems', 'sleep disorders', 'habit disorders' and 'backwardness' (Williams 1938: 145–8). Of all these only 'backwardness' did not necessarily present a problem to be remedied. The backward child might become maladjusted if badly managed and placed in an environment that was too challenging. Other children, whether their presenting problem was 'thumbsucking', 'day-dreaming' or 'cruelty', were all exhibiting 'the danger signs of faulty adjustment', with the remedy lying in the modification of the child's environment, including the human environment, and in a retraining of the child into more appropriate responses. Conduct which at the beginning of the decade was regarded as the outward sign of an inner disturbance requiring diagnosis and individual treatment was by the end of the 1930s repositioned as the problem of maladjustment: a problem which might display itself in different ways, but could (potentially at least) be remedied by a common set of strategies. Further, according to Williams, the best assistance that the medical profession could offer the 'pre-school child' was in educating parents about the reasons for maladjustment and 'aiding in every way the extension of nursery schools and kindergartens'.

GENDER AND TEMPERAMENT

Given the preceding analysis, it ought come as no surprise that, in the Australian context, the first registration of disparities between males and females in meeting the challenges of development occurred in the modest surroundings of the Collingwood Demonstration Centre, in an investigation conducted not by a child psychologist but by May Gutteridge, Kindergarten Director. Admittedly, our investigation may have made the drawing of boundaries between the psychologist and kindergarten worker and their fields of expertise, at least in the recent past, appear somewhat arbitrary: if so, part of the purpose of mounting a history of the formation of the present problem posed by the ATP will have been achieved.

Gutteridge's registration of differences between male and female children appeared in the context of an investigation into the duration of attention spans in the Collingwood children conducted during 1935 (Gutteridge 1935). The objective was to determine whether the ability to attend to a task increased with age. She was able to conclude:

> laziness, idleness and inattention are deviations from the normal curve of growth in the habit of attending. They can therefore be classed as 'bad habits' and as such they are preventable, and with special study into the causes in individual cases, they should be remediable.
>
> (Gutteridge 1935: 46)

The possible influence of sex on attention spans was readily calculable. Gutteridge had only two variables to work with, and the task of working out averages for boys and girls was a matter of simple arithmetic. The population of girls revealed consistently longer attention spans, with a clear acceleration over boys taking place between the ages of 4 and 5 (Gutteridge 1935: 32). But it was one matter to establish that there was a difference, and another to work out what the significance of that difference might be. Gutteridge suggested that further research was needed before it could be firmly concluded that the difference was 'genuine', and whether its presence indicated a need for an adjustment of the environment the nursery school provided for boys.

Gutteridge then, in 1935, appears poised on the brink of discovering that boys were more likely than girls to display 'bad habits', and thus could properly be regarded as a problem population sixty years in advance of the ATP. But to draw this conclusion would be to once again confer stability onto the child as an object of study, and to assume that the 'nature' of boys and girls exists in an essential underlying form that child psychologists, or those with other claims to expertise, may variously recognise, misrecognise, represent or misrepresent. Moreover, it would require assuming that the presence or absence in child populations of those attributes which happen to be valued by a range of authorities is simply a matter of chance: that the appearance of the 'habit of attending', for example, has nothing to do with the child's exposure to an expertly organised educational milieu designed to maximise this capacity.

Gutteridge's hesitation over whether the difference was 'genuine', a registration of inherent differences between males and females, or an outcome of differences in the environmental mileu experienced by males and females is worth attending to. Margot Prior, the ATP project leader, is similarly hesitant on judging whether the difference in the achievement of the valued attribute of self-regulation is a product of nature or parental training (Heath 1995: 4). Nor, she suggests, can there be any expectation that this epistemological uncertainty will ever be adequately resolved. But this is no impediment to advising on the reorganisation of domestic and educational environments in ways designed to enhance the production of this quality amongst all children, and amongst 'boys' in particular. Gutteridge too, given that attention spans correlated positively with other valued traits like alertness and dependability, set about altering the nursery school/kindergarten milieu (more cooperative, less teacher-directed work and play) and making recommendations for changes at home (the provision of play materials that held attention, mother in the background). Like Prior, Gutteridge was reasoning in terms of risk: acting on attention was a preventive strategy against the development of other problems (Castel 1991).

CONCLUSION

Historical investigations suggest that the elements that go to make up the 'competent' child are not stable over time, and that the constituents of competence are contingent upon institutional objectives. But they also suggest that current realities should not be understood as the outcome of a mere shifting of the goal posts on an otherwise stable playing field of human attributes permanently fixed to sexed bodies. We ought, in other words, to expect that the self-regulation gap currently registered between male and female children will be narrowed, and that further disparities between different populations of children will continue to be identified and worked upon. But what we ought not to expect is that child psychology will clear up its epistemological uncertainties, or abandon its technical expertise in the management of child populations.

The ATP's casting of boys as a population at risk of maladjustment owes nothing to discoveries of the inner workings of the human mind, and a great deal to techniques of governing child populations, including those which have enabled the identification of problem populations as the necessary prior step to the development of strategies for their modification. Presumably, few would wish to claim that at the current moment aggression ought be positively rather than negatively valued. Rather than posing the ATP as hostile to the efforts to garner scarce resources for girls' education, the current problematising of aggression in educational milieux may be more usefully understood as an outcome of the efforts and programmes mounted by feminist educators and mental health workers to change the ways in which the conduct of males and females is thought about and responded to: an outcome of the constitution of gender as a problem. In the 1970s and 1980s, on the other hand, child psychology lent its expertise to the resolution of a different gender trouble surfacing in schools: girls' low participation rates and performance in the key curricular areas of maths, science and technology. That the competent child cited by Walkerdine – active, enquiring, autonomous – performed well in the maths classroom says little about the existence of an underlying nature of boys and girls, but rather more about the institutional surfaces of emergence of those questions which child psychology has made its own.

Ten years into the largest investigation of temperament ever undertaken, the leaders of the ATP are prepared to concede that many of the epistemological questions surrounding temperament remain opaque. The theory that temperament is 'hard-wired' into the personality, for example, is slightly at odds with the finding that the mass of children are rated differently at different times, although the extremes at each end of the conduct scale show more consistency (Prior 1992: 97–9; Sanson *et al.* 1990: 179–92). On the other hand this suggests that 'environmental modification' will be a suitable response to manifestations of difficult behaviour on the part of the ordinary child (Prior 1992: 105). Further research can be expected to cast more light on these puzzling aspects of temperament. But the value of temperament as a predictor of future conduct is clear:

> Despite the fact that we cannot specify 'what it is', we know quite a lot about 'what it does'. . . . Temperament in and of itself is not so important as the match or mismatch between the individual's temperament and his environment. . . . There is a steadily increasing number of studies which report on the relationships between temperament and a variety of outcomes including behaviour disorder, adjustment to school, adjustment to family break-up, to medical conditions, to parental pathology, and adult adjustment.
>
> (Prior 1992: 95–7)

The temperament project couches its larger ambitions in terms of discovering more about temperament, discovering more about a cloudy and contested facet of what makes people behave in certain ways. But, if at the project's end 'what it is' remains as opaque as at the outset, there will be no failure. Rather, a great deal more will be known about 'what it does', and how 'it' might be acted upon to transform children at risk of maladjustment into more competent children. You do not, as it were, have to know quite what you are dealing with to have the know-how to deal with it.

REFERENCES

Campbell, A.W. (1935) 'Psychoses of adolescence', *Medical Journal of Australia*, 12 October: 479.

Castel, R. (1991) 'From dangerousness to risk', in G. Burchell, C. Gordon and P. Miller (eds) *The Foucault Effect, Studies in Governmentality*, Hemel Hempstead: Harvester Wheatsheaf.

Cunningham, K.S. (1932) 'Problem children in Melbourne schools', *Australian Education Studies (First Series)*, Melbourne: Melbourne University Press.

Dawson, W.S. (1935) 'Psychoses of adolescence', *Medical Journal of Australia*, 12 October: 478–9.

Farran-Ridge, C. (1935) 'Psychoses of adolescence', *Medical Journal of Australia*, 12 October: 479.

Foucault, M. (1976) 'On governmentality', *Ideology & Consciousness*, 6: 5–21.

Foucault, M. (1977) 'Nietzsche, genealogy, history', in D. Bouchard (ed.), *Language, Counter-Memory, Practice*, Ithaca: Cornell University Press.

Foucault, M. (1981) 'Questions of method: an interview with Michel Foucault', *Ideology & Consciousness*, 8: 4–14.

Foucault, M. (1988) 'Technologies of the self', in L.H. Martin, H. Gutman and P.H. Hutton (eds) *Technologies of the Self, A Seminar with Michel Foucault*, Cambridge, Massachusetts: University of Massachusetts Press.

Gutteridge, M.V. (1932) 'The story of an Australian nursery school', *Australian Education Studies (First Series)*, Melbourne: Melbourne University Press.

Gutteridge, M.V. (1935) *The Duration of Attention in Young Children*, Educational Research Series no. 41, Melbourne: Melbourne University Press.

Heath, S. (1995) 'Easygoing children find life easier', *The Age*, 6 December: 4.

Legge, K. (1995) 'Boy have we got trouble', *Australian Magazine*, 11–12 March: 26–31.

Lush, M. (1926) *Progressive Kindergarten Methods*, Melbourne: Lothian Press.

Prior, M. (1989) 'The Australian Temperament Project', in G.A. Kohnstamm, J.E. Bates and M.K. Rothbart (eds) *Temperament in Childhood*, Chichester: John Wiley and Sons.

Prior, M. (1992) 'Development of temperament', in P.C. Heaven (ed.) *Life-span Development*, Marrickville: Harcourt Brace Jovanovich.

Riley, D. (1988) *'Am I That Name?' Feminism and the Category of Women in History*, London: Macmillan.

Rose, N. (1985) *The Psychological Complex: Psychology, Politics and Society in England 1869-1939*, London: Routledge and Kegan Paul.

Rose, N. (1988) 'Calculable minds and manageable individuals', *History of the Human Sciences*, 1, 2: 179–200.

Rose, N. (1989) *Governing the Soul. The Shaping of the Private Self*, London: Routledge.

Sanson, A., Prior, M. and Kyrios, M. (1990) 'Contamination of measures in temperament research', *Merrill-Palmer Quarterly*, 36, 2: 179–92.

Sanson, A., Prior, M., Smart, D. and Oberklaid, F. (1993) 'Gender differences in aggression in childhood: implications for a peaceful world', *Australian Psychologist*, 28, 2: 86–92.

Sweet, M. (1995) 'Boys: sadder and badder than girls', *Sydney Morning Herald*, 5 April: 1.

Tyler, D. (1993) 'Making better children', in D. Meredyth and D. Tyler (eds) *Child and Citizen, Genealogies of Schooling and Subjectivity*, Brisbane: Institute of Cultural Policy Studies.

Walkerdine, V. (1985) 'On the regulation of speaking and silence: subjectivity, class and gender in contemporary schooling', in C. Steedman, C. Urwin and V. Walkerdine (eds) *Language, Gender and Childhood*, London: Routledge and Kegan Paul.

Williams, J.F. (1932) 'Child guidance work in a public hospital', *Medical Journal of Australia*, 3 September: 294–9.

Williams, J.F. (1935) 'Psychoses of adolescence', *Medical Journal of Australia*, 12 October: 480.

Williams, J.F. (1938) 'Mental hygiene of the pre-school child', *Medical Journal of Australia*, 30 July: 145–8.

Chapter 5

Foucault and the medicalisation critique

Deborah Lupton

INTRODUCTION

Since the 1970s, a perspective that may loosely be termed 'the medicalisation critique' has been a central stance in sociological writings on the medical profession. In this chapter, I interrogate the notion of medicalisation and explore the ways that a Foucauldian perspective may contribute to understandings of power in relation to medical knowledge and practice and the medical encounter. I argue that the writings of Foucault and his followers, while not necessarily using the term 'medicalisation' or adhering to the versions of power relations usually presented by proponents of the orthodox medicalisation critique, tend to present a consonant vision of a world in which individuals' lives are profoundly experienced and understood through the discourses and practices of medicine and its allied professions.

While the Foucauldian perspective articulates a more complex notion of the role played by medicine in contemporary Western societies than is generally put forward by proponents of the orthodox medicalisation critique, this perspective itself is characterised by some confusions, difficulties, obscurities and gaps. Any discussion of the ways that Foucault's work has been used in relation to the medicalisation thesis becomes complicated by the fact that his *oeuvre* itself encompassed a number of shifts and inconsistencies over time, as well as a certain (perhaps deliberate) lack of clarity in the ways in which he described power relations and their outcome. This is reflected in the work of others who have used Foucault's writings to theorise the social relations of medicine and health in Western societies. One major problem is the tendency of Foucault and those using his work to neglect examination of the ways that hegemonic medical discourses and practices are variously taken up, negotiated or transformed by members of the lay population in their quest to maximise their health status and avoid physical distress and pain. It is here that a Foucauldian perspective has had little to offer hitherto. However, I would argue that insights derived from a phenomenology informed by Foucault's later work on the practices of the self may go some way to meet this lacuna.

THE ORTHODOX MEDICALISATION CRITIQUE

The medicalisation critique, as it has taken shape in the sociological literature, arose initially from Marxist perspectives and the liberal humanism that underlay the emergence of social movements in the 1960s and 1970s. These approaches were characterised by their emphasis on the importance of individual freedom, human rights and social change. Their critique of the ways that society is structured included calling into question the social role played by members of powerful and high-status occupational groups such as the legal and medical professions. At least in part, the medicalisation critique was a repudiation of the Parsonian structural functionalism that dominated medical sociology in the 1950s and early 1960s and was viewed by its critics as being overly politically conservative and supportive of medical authority. Gerhardt (1989: xxv) traces the origin of the medicalisation critique from the time of the student revolutions in Europe in 1968, when medical sociologists were stimulated into realising that 'justice and inequality were legitimate topics for academic enquiry'. Many medical sociologists took up this critique in their own professional work, seeking to challenge and subvert the power of the medical profession.

Supporters of the medicalisation critique have generally identified a central paradox: medicine, as it is practised in Western societies, despite its alleged lack of effectiveness in treating a wide range of conditions and its iatrogenic side-effects, has increasingly amassed power and influence. They contend that social life and social problems had become more and more 'medicalised', or viewed through the prism of scientific medicine as 'diseases'. Critics such as Irving Zola (1972) and Eliot Freidson (1970) argued that medicine had begun to take on the role of social regulation traditionally performed by religion and the law. One of the most vociferous advocates of the medicalisation critique was Ivan Illich (1975), who contended that rather than improving people's health, contemporary scientific medicine under-mined it, both through the side-effects of medical treatment and by diminishing lay people's capacity for autonomy in dealing with their own health care.

The notion that individuals should not have their autonomy constrained by more powerful others is central to the ideals of the medicalisation critique. In concert with liberal humanist ideals, critics argue that becoming 'medicalised' denies rational, independent human action by allowing members of an authoritative group (in this case the medical profession) to dictate to others how they should behave. There is a concern evident in the literature on medicalisation about the 'dependency' that contemporary scientific medicine is seen to encourage. As this would suggest, the term 'medicalisation' is generally used in the sociological literature in a pejorative manner: to be 'medicalised' is never a desirable state of being. As such, 'medicalisation' is positioned as something which should resisted, in favour of some degree of 'de-medicalisation'. Proponents of the critique generally take an overwhelmingly negative view of members of the medical profession, seeing doctors as attempting to enhance their position by presenting themselves as possessing the exclusive right to define and treat illness, thereby subordinating the opinions and knowledges of lay people. This increasing power of scientific medicine, it is contended, has detrimental effects for traditionally disempowered and exploited social groups by deflecting questions of social inequality into the realm of illness and disease, there to be treated inappropriately by drugs and other medical therapies.

Proponents of the medicalisation critique call attention to the notion that patients in general, because of their lack of medical knowledge, are placed in the position of vulnerable supplicants when they seek the attention of doctors, with consequently little opportunity to challenge doctors' decisions. This is particularly the case, they argue, for members of the working class and other socio-economically disadvantaged groups, whose lack of power is further entrenched through their interactions with powerful doctors who seek to maintain the social status quo. Research carried out exploring the doctor–patient relationship from this perspective has tended to focus on the ways that the medical consultation facilitates the power of doctors over patients and supports capitalist ideologies. For example, in his analysis of the 'micro-politics of medicine', the Marxist sociologist Howard Waitzkin (1984) looked at the verbal encounters between doctors and patients with the intention of identifying the features of the encounter that 'medicalise' and 'depoliticise' the social structural dimensions of ill health. Waitzkin argued that 'The medical encounter is one arena where the dominant ideologies of a society are reinforced and where individuals' acquiescence is sought' (1984: 339). In addition to those writers interested in class struggle, the medicalisation critique has been taken up with enthusiasm by feminist critics of medicine (for example, Ehrenreich and English 1974). Feminist critics have viewed the medical profession as a largely patriarchal institution that used definitions of illness and disease to maintain the relative inequality of women by drawing attention to their weakness and susceptibility to illness and by taking control over areas of women's lives such as pregnancy and childbirth that were previously the domain of female lay practitioners and midwives.

The answers to medicalisation, according to most critics, include challenging the right of medicine to make claims about its powers to define and treat illness and disease and encouraging the state to exert greater regulation over the actions of the medical profession so as to limit its expansion and 'deprofessionalise' it. Most critics also advocate the 'empowerment' of patients (often renamed 'consumers'), encouraging people to 'take back control' over their own health by engaging in preventive health activities, assuming the role of 'consumer' by challenging the decisions and knowledge of doctors in the medical encounter, joining patient advocacy groups and eschewing medicine by seeking the attentions of alternative practitioners.

The medicalisation critique was one of the most dominant perspectives in the sociology of health and illness in the 1970s and into the 1980s. It remains a dominant approach in the 1990s, particularly for feminist writers, those critics who still adhere to a Marxist perspective on health and illness and proponents of the consumerist approach to medicine. There is no doubt that the medicalisation critique represented an important shift in thinking among medical sociologists in calling attention to the possibility for inequity in medical encounters and the delivery of health care. Nonetheless, the critique may itself be criticised on a number of grounds. One major difficulty with the orthodox medicalisation critique is its rather black-and-white portrayal of Western medicine as largely detracting from rather than improving people's health status, of doctors as intent on increasing their power over their patients rather than seeking to help them, and of patients as largely helpless, passive and disempowered, their agency crushed beneath the might of the medical profession. Indeed, in much of this literature, 'The asymmetry of the relationship is exaggerated to the point that the lay client becomes not the beneficiary but the *victim* of the consultation' (Atkinson 1995: 33, original emphasis).

In their efforts to denounce medicine and to represent doctors as oppressive forces, orthodox critics tend to display little recognition of the ways that it may contribute to good health, the relief of pain and the recovery from illness, or the value that many people understandably place on these outcomes. They also fail to acknowledge the ambivalent nature of the feelings and opinions that many people have in relation to medicine, or the ways that patients willingly participate in medical dominance and may indeed seek 'medicalisation'. As de Swaan has pointed out, the power of the professions to make judgements about normality must involve complicity on the part of their clients, students, charges or patients. This complicity inevitably incorporates latent conflict and resistances, 'a shifting balance between manifest collaboration and tacit opposition in the relations between those who come for help and those who profess to provide it' (de Swaan 1990: 1). Rather than there being a struggle for power between the dominant party (doctors) and the less powerful party (patients), there is collusion between the two to reproduce medical dominance.

FOUCAULT AND MEDICALISATION

The gradual entry of Foucault's writings into Anglophone medical sociology over the past fifteen years or so (albeit more so in Australia and Britain than in North America) has also challenged some of the central assumptions of the orthodox medicalisation critique, particularly in relation to its conceptualisation of power and medical knowledge. Foucault's writings emphasise the positive and productive rather than the repressive nature of power. Indeed, Foucault argued, the very seductiveness of power in modern societies is that it is productive rather than simply confining:

> what makes power hold good, what makes it accepted, is simply the fact that it doesn't only weigh on us as a force that says no, but that it traverses and produces things, it induces pleasure, forms knowledge, produces discourse. It needs to be considered as a productive network which runs through the whole social body, much more than as a negative instance whose function is repression.
>
> (Foucault 1984a: 61)

Here the important feature of medical knowledge and practice is their participation in the very constitution of bodies and subjectivities. In *The Birth of the Clinic* (1975), Foucault argues that, over time, various medical paradigms have provided important systems of knowledge and related practices by which we have not only understood but also experienced our bodies. From this perspective, medical power may be viewed as the underlying resource by which diseases and illnesses are identified and dealt with. This perspective fits into the broader social constructionist approach in understanding medical knowledge not simply as a given and objective set of 'facts' but as a belief system shaped through social and political relations. Most writers adopting the orthodox medicalisation critique would be broadly sympathetic to such an approach, particularly in their arguments that medicine tends to transform social issues into 'diseases'. Where a Foucauldian perspective largely departs from the usual approach is by going somewhat further in contending that there is no such thing as an 'authentic' human body that exists outside medical discourse and practice. Rather, the body and its various parts are understood as constructed through discourses and practices, through the 'clinical gaze' exerted by medical practitioners. Thus, 'A body analysed for humours contains humours; a body analysed for organs and tissues is constituted by organs and tissues; a body analysed for psychosocial functioning is a psychosocial object' (Armstrong 1994: 25).

From the Foucauldian perspective, power as it operates in the medical encounter is a disciplinary power that provides guidelines about how patients should understand, regulate and experience their bodies. The central strategies of disciplinary power are observation, examination, measurement and the comparison of individuals against an established norm, bringing them into a field of visibility. It is exercised not primarily through direct coercion or violence (although it must be emphasised that these strategies are still used from time to time), but rather through persuading its subjects that certain ways of behaving and thinking are appropriate for them. The power that doctors have in relation to patients, therefore, might be thought of as a facilitating capacity or resource, a means of bringing into being the subjects 'doctor' and 'patient' and the phenomenon of the patient's 'illness'. From this perspective, doctors are not considered to be 'figures of domination', but rather 'links in a set of power relations', 'people through whom power passe[s] or who are important in the field of power relations' (Foucault 1984b: 247). Unlike those who assert the orthodox medicalisation critique, a Foucauldian perspective argues, therefore, that it is impossible to remove power from members of the medical profession and hand it over to patients. Power is not a possession of particular social groups, but is relational, a strategy which is invested in and transmitted through all social groups. This more complex view of power goes some way to recognising the collusive nature of power relations in relation to medicine.

Another important dimension of the Foucauldian understanding of power in the medical context is an emphasis on the dispersed nature of power, its lack of a central political rationale. Proponents of the orthodox medicalisation thesis tend to view members of the medical profession as consciously seeking to gain power and status and limit other groups' power, largely by eliciting the state's support. In contrast, Foucauldian scholars tend to argue that the clinical gaze is not intentional in terms of originating from a particular type of group seeking domination over others. There is not a single medicine but a series of loosely linked assemblages, each with different rationalities (Osborne 1994: 42). Foucault and his followers have emphasised that the fields and concerns of medicine are diverse and heterogeneous, taking place at sites such as workplaces, schools, supermarkets and homes as well as the clinic, hospital or surgery. The state is, of course, involved in the reproduction of medical dominance, including regulating the conditions for the licensing of medical practitioners, but there are also other agencies and institutions involved beyond the state, and indeed the interests of the medical profession and those of the state often clash. (This can be seen in the continual battles between doctors' lobby groups such as the Australian Medical Association and the government ministers who hold the responsibility for the administration of health portfolios.)

All this is not to argue that Foucault and his followers would necessarily dispute the notion that contemporary societies are subject to great influence from scientific medicine. Quite the contrary: while they may not use the term 'medicalisation', one of their central contentions is that society is medicalised in a profound way, serving to monitor and administer the bodies of citizens in an effort to regulate and maintain social order as well as promoting good health and productivity. Medical knowledge and practice serve to differentiate between social groups, to identify and propose means of addressing inequities in health and social advantage. Medicine and health have become central to the notion of the 'normal' person because, in part, medicine:

> has come to link the ethical question of how we should behave to the scientific question of who we truly are and what our nature is as human beings, as life forms in a living system, as simultaneously unique individuals and constituents of a population.
>
> (Rose 1994: 67–8)

Medicalisation is evident in the ways in which warnings about health risks have become common events. People are constantly urged to conduct their everyday lives in order to avoid potential disease or early death. As a result, 'Sociologically speaking, everyone lives under the medical regime, a light regime for those who are not yet patients, stricter according to how dependent on doctors one becomes' (de Swaan 1990: 57). This is particularly the case for older people and the chronically ill, in relation to improvements in longevity and medical treatment for acute illnesses. Where once, for instance, physical activity might have been undertaken for the purposes of 'character formation', 'experiencing nature' or 'the pleasure of functioning', it is now often understood as a medical activity, undertaken for the purposes of good health (de Swaan 1990: 59).

CRITIQUES OF THE FOUCAULDIAN PERSPECTIVE

One feature of Foucauldian writings on medicine that has been the subject of quite some criticism is their general focus on analysing the discourses evident in official texts and their neglect of the ways that medical practitioners and lay people themselves practise and experience medicine. In relation to this criticism, Foucault and his followers have also been brought to task for the deterministic nature of their argument, in which discourses are represented as subjugating human agency with little scope for resistance or acknowledgement of the 'lived experience' of the body. This is particularly evident in the concept of the 'docile body' of the patient caught in the clinical gaze, which tends to echo the negative view of medicine articulated by the orthodox medicalisation critics. Writers in this vein have tended to focus on surveillance and medical domination, and the inability of the patient to return the clinical gaze. They often represent medical power as overwhelmingly coercive and confining, despite Foucault's own insistence about the productive rather than repressive nature of power. Indeed, at its most extreme, the conception of power as 'everywhere', as an inevitable element of knowledge and as constitutive of reality, tends to suggest the individuals are enmeshed in a sticky web of medical power from which they will never be able to emerge, their struggles only further imprisoning them.

Those writers who have focused on the 'docile body' have drawn mainly on such works as *The Birth of the Clinic* (1975), *Madness and Civilization* (1967) and *Discipline and Punish* (1977). Their subsequent representation of medical power is perhaps not surprising, given that these histories are replete with vivid descriptions of the oppressed and tortured bodies of the ill, the mad or the criminal and efforts to render these bodies knowable, docile and productive (see, for example, the opening pages of *The Birth of the Clinic*). This approach is evident in the work of Foucauldians such as David Armstrong, whose influential *Political Anatomy of the Body* (1983) and other writings (for example, Armstrong 1984, 1987) tend to portray patients as passive bodies in the grip of the ever-more powerful discourses and practices of panoptic medicine:

> The prisoner in the Panopticon and the patient at the end of the stethoscope, both remain silent as the techniques of surveillance sweep over them. They know they are being monitored but they remain unaware of what has been seen or what has been heard.
>
> (Armstrong 1987: 70)

Foucault himself was careful to emphasise frequently that where there is power there are always resistances, for power inevitably creates and works through resistance. He acknowledged that the existence of strategies of power does not necessarily correspond with the successful exertion of power, and that intended outcomes often fail to materialise because disciplinary strategies break down or fail. This is as true of the practice of medicine as of any other field of power. As May has stated in relation to the medical context, there is 'a massive array of practical problems which actors operating in medical (and other) settings encounter as they attempt to monitor subjects' (1992: 486; see also Porter 1996). Rather than being interested in power as an ideology, as is the concern of Marxist critiques, Foucault commented in an interview that he was interested in 'the question of the body and the effects of power on it' (Foucault 1980: 58). Frustratingly enough, however, Foucault's concept of resistance was never really explained in detail. Instead, he made various somewhat elliptical comments about the interrelationship of power, embodiment and resistance, such as the statement: 'Power, after investing itself in the body, finds itself exposed to a counter-attack in the same body' (Foucault 1980: 56).

There is somewhat of a disjuncture, therefore, between Foucault's notion of the 'docile body' and his recognition of resistance at the local sites at which power operates and the inevitability of the failure of disciplinary and surveillance strategies directed at the patient. This confusion is reflected in some of the work of those scholars who have used Foucault's writings to comment on medical power. In their focus on the disciplinary regimes and apparatuses that surround the body in the medical or institutional context, there is little discussion in many Foucauldian accounts of the phenomenological body, or how people respond to the external discourses and strategies that attempt to discipline them. Nor is there much discussion of how these responses are mediated through such factors as gender, age, social class, sexual identity and ethnicity. While it is clearly important to trace the discourses and practices of medicine and to demonstrate shifts as well as continuities over time, it is equally important to attempt to investigate empirically the ways that members of the lay population respond to the clinical gaze, to 'bring them alive' rather than represent them simply as docile or passive bodies constrained at every turn by hegemonic discourses. As Chris Shilling contends:

> it is necessary to allow for lived experience, for the *phenomenology* of the body. Bodies may be surrounded by and perceived through discourses, but they are *irreducible* to discourse. The body needs to be grasped as an actual material phenomenon which is both affected by and *affects* knowledge and society.
>
> (1991: 664, emphases in the original)

In Foucault's later work, such as volume three of *The History of Sexuality* (1986), he began to move away from the notion of power as operating on individuals via dominating institutions to speculate on the modes of the formation of personhood, or, as he termed it, the technology or practices of the self. As he commented in an interview,

> Perhaps I've insisted too much on the technology of domination and power. I am more and more interested in the interaction between oneself and others and in the technologies of individual domination, the history of how an individual acts upon himself [sic], in the technology of self.
>
> (1988: 146)

Central to this new emphasis on the self-discipline is a focus on the interrelationship between the imperatives of bodily management expressed at the institutional level and ways that individuals engage in the conduct of everyday life. Foucault articulated an interest in the local techniques and strategies of power, or the micro-powers that are exercised at the level of everyday life, and the ways that resistance may be generated at those levels by people refusing to engage in these techniques and strategies. In other words, he was beginning to devote attention to the phenomenology of power relations. Foucault's work on this project was cut short due to his death, and this theorising therefore remained underdeveloped. Nonetheless, this turn towards the ontology of experience, moving towards a phenomenology of everyday life and subjectivity, provides a means of addressing the ways that the so-called 'docile' body of the patient may, at least on some occasions, resist docility as part of self-formation. Such a project draws upon Foucault's own intention in his work to identify 'subjugated knowledges', or those knowledges that tend to be buried and disguised beneath more dominant, often more 'scientific' or 'expert' knowledges.

Those few researchers in medical sociology who have attempted to use a Foucauldian theoretical framework to analyse empirical data derived from interviews with lay people have demonstrated the diversity of responses to the strategies of medical power and the contradictions and conflicts that exist in the ways that people respond to doctors. One instructive example is a study by Bloor and McIntosh (1990). They interviewed Scottish mothers receiving home visits from health visitors and used the method of participant observation to record the ways that members of four therapeutic communities responded to the external strategies of medical power that attempted to shape their behaviour through surveillance. Bloor and McIntosh noted that the subjects of the surveying therapeutic gaze responded in various ways, including direct rejection and attack on the value and legitimacy of the health workers' attentions, non-cooperation, silence, escape, avoidance and, most commonly of all, concealment. The mothers, for example, would simply not tell the health workers about some of their actions, or would lie to them when directly asked.

Sociological accounts often fail to acknowledge the interpersonal aspects of the medical encounter, the mutual dependencies that doctors and patients have upon each other and the emotions and desires that motivate behaviour. In my own recent empirical research using interviews with both lay people and medical practitioners in Sydney (see Lupton forthcoming), the data suggested that the medical encounter involves a continual negotiation of power that is contingent upon the context in which the patient interacts with the doctor. Such factors as the type of medical complaint, the age, ethnicity and gender of the patient and doctor, emotional dimensions and the patient's accumulated embodied experiences all shaped the encounter in diverse ways. In their interviews, patients said that at times they sought to dominate their doctor, to adopt explicitly consumerist positions, sometimes directly expressing hostility and anger. At other times, they were apparently quite happy to give themselves over to the doctor without question. Indeed, this study found that the majority of lay people interviewed continued to want to invest their trust and faith in their doctor, and welcomed the doctor showing an interest in their lives, including their personal lives. For those people who had experienced serious illness or hospitalisation, it was vital that they felt they could rely upon their doctors. This investment of trust and faith, however, is also problematic for many people, because it means relinquishing some degree of autonomy, allowing oneself to become dependent upon another and exposing one's body, feelings and innermost thoughts to another. In the relationship between carer and cared-for, there is a continual tension on the part of the cared-for between wanting and appreciating care and resenting it (Fox 1995; Lupton forthcoming).

Foucault's notion of the practices of the self can be brought into play to analyse the ways that people respond to the medical encounter. The doctor–patient relationship is a central site at which subjugated knowledges and the practices of the self play a major role in the interrelation of institutional and localised power. When consulting a doctor, individuals may, on at least some occasions, and if they so choose, attempt to struggle against, challenge or subvert those disciplinary techniques they experience as restricting of their autonomy. That patients often fail to take 'doctors' orders' is evident in the extensive medical literature on the problem of patient compliance with medical regimens. On the other hand, those individuals who 'go along' with medical advice need not necessarily be viewed as passively accepting the orders of the doctor or the medical gaze, but rather could be seen as engaging in practices of the self that they consider are vital to their own well-being and freedom from discomfort or pain. As the above research suggests, individuals may constitute themselves as ideal-type 'consumers' as part of the presentation of the self as an autonomous, reflexive individual who refuses to take a passive, orthodox patient role. Alternatively they may present themselves as someone who 'follows doctor's orders', who is a 'good patient', working actively in the medical encounter to achieve this. Sometimes they may pursue both types of subject position simultaneously or variously. In each case, the individual has a personal, emotional investment in presenting her- or himself in a certain manner, as a certain 'type of person' engaged in 'rational' and 'civilized' behaviour consonant with her or his social or embodied position at the time.

The notion of the practices of the self, however, suggests an actor who is always consciously aware of what she or he is doing, who is engaging in a reflexive evaluation of the situation and responding accordingly to maximise her or his life changes, who approaches life as if it were a rational enterprise. There needs to be a recognition that human motivation also originates from the unconscious. At a less conscious or 'irrational' level, patients may behave in assertive or hostile ways because of their very dependence on doctors, splitting off their fears and anxieties about their pain or illness and projecting them onto the doctor. Or they may willingly engage in a relationship with their doctor that echoes the parent–child relationship, because of the emotional comfort that offers (Stein 1985). Post-structuralist theory has posited a notion of subjectivity that incorporates acknowledgement of the inevitably fragmented self, the contradictory self that is pulled between a number of desires emerging from both the unconscious and the conscious (Henriques *et al.* 1984). This concept of the self recognises the emotional investments people make in their relations with others, the ways in which different sources of the self intertwine and become important at different times for the same person. In this conceptualisation, subjectivity may be understood as dynamic and contextual rather than static, and as often fraught with ambivalence, irrationality and conflict. It is this recognition of the continual ambivalence of subjectivity that may provide some insights into the ways that people are often complicit in the reproduction of medical power as well as frequently seeking to challenge it.

CONCLUSION

This chapter has shown that both significant similarities and differences between the orthodox medicalisation critique and Foucauldian commentaries on scientific medicine may be identified. In broad terms, both approaches agree that medicine is a dominant institution that in Western societies has come to play an increasingly important role in everyday life, shaping the ways that we think about and live our bodies. There is less agreement, however, on how detrimental this state of affairs is for members of the lay population and what kinds of action are required in response. For orthodox critics, I have argued, medicalisation is typically represented as negative, a repressive and coercive process that limits the autonomy and encourages the dependency of lay people. Advocates of this critique therefore routinely call for strategies for 'de-medicalising' that are assumed to improve the lot of lay people. Because orthodox critics generally have embraced a liberal humanist political position and a view of power as a property of social groups, they continue to argue for the possibility that medical power may be diminished in favour of greater autonomy on the part of lay people.

Some Foucauldians seek to critique (even if implicitly rather than explicitly) the expansion of the 'clinical gaze' in ways that echo the orthodox medicalisation critics. However, most writers who have been influenced by Foucault, in their awareness of the contradictions and naiveties inherent in calls for 'de-medicalisation', tend to be more equivocal about proposing actual strategies for changing medical practice that go beyond deconstructing dominant discourses and identifying 'subjugated knowledges'. From the Foucauldian perspective there are a number of inconsistencies and paradoxes that may be identified in the orthodox medicalisation critique. One difficulty is the kinds of solutions that tend to be offered. Those who argue that lay people should become more informed about medical matters, so as to 'take control' from doctors, may be regarded as paradoxically advocating a greater 'medicalisation' of people's lives by encouraging them to acquire medical knowledge for themselves more actively. Encouraging individuals to engage in preventive health activities possibly avoids one form of 'medicalisation' (clinical). On the other hand, it takes up another form (preventive medicine and 'self-care') that moves medical and health concerns into every corner of everyday life, including diet, physical exercise, sleep patterns and relationships with others. So too, a Foucauldian critique may argue that alternative therapies often level a much more intense and individualistic gaze at the relationship of people's everyday activities and their private lives with their health status than does medicine. Thus the move towards 'de-medicalisation' may be interpreted paradoxically as a growing penetration of the clinical gaze into the everyday lives of citizens, including their emotional states, the nature of their interpersonal relationships, their management of 'stress' and their 'lifestyle' choices.

Further, the Foucauldian understanding of subjectivity and the body as partly constructed *through* medical discourses and practices calls into question the assumption of the orthodox medicalisation critics that 'de-medicalisation' is a source of freedom and greater autonomy for lay people. The Foucauldian perspective would argue that it is not simply a matter of stripping away medicine as a dominant frame of reference to reveal the 'true' body, as most of the orthodox critics would argue. From the Foucauldian perspective, 'de-medicalising' the body, or viewing it through alternative frames of reference that are not medical, may well lead to different, but not more 'authentic' modes of subjectivity and embodiment.

Given the complexities that have been raised by the Foucauldian critique, it may seem difficult to take a position on the issue of 'medicalisation'. I would argue, however, that the awareness of these difficulties is itself an important outcome that has emerged from the entrée of Foucauldian perspectives into the debate. One possibility I have identified in furthering the insights offered by Foucauldian perspectives is taking up Foucault's later interest in the practices of the self and engaging in a phenomenological analysis of the experiences people have in the context of medical care. Neither the orthodox medicalisation critique nor the Foucauldian perspective has adequately taken account of the mutual dependencies and the emotional and psychodynamic dimensions of the medical encounter, preferring to rely upon a notion of the rational actor. Yet, as I argued, a recognition of the 'irrational' and contradictory aspects of the relationship that lay people have with members of the medical profession goes some way to explaining why it is that 'power, after investing itself in the body, finds itself exposed to a counter-attack in the same body'. It remains for scholars and researchers to devote more attention to the ways that the discourses on the human body, medicine and health care that may be identified in such sites as the mass media, medical and public health literature and policy documents are recognised, ignored, contested, translated and transformed in the context of everyday experience.

ACKNOWLEDGEMENT

This chapter was written as part of series of papers emerging from a study on patients' and medical practitioners' views on the medical profession and the coverage of the medical profession in the mass media funded by a large grant from the Australian Research Council in 1994–5.

REFERENCES

Armstrong, D. (1983) *Political Anatomy of the Body: Medical Knowledge in Britain in the Twentieth Century*, Cambridge: Cambridge University Press.
Armstrong, D. (1984) 'The patient's view', *Social Science and Medicine*, 18, 9: 737–44.
Armstrong, D. (1987) 'Bodies of knowledge: Foucault and the problem of human anatomy', in G. Scambler (ed.) *Sociological Theory and Medical Sociology*, London: Tavistock.
Armstrong, D. (1994) 'Bodies of knowledge/knowledge of bodies', in C. Jones and R. Porter (eds) *Reassessing Foucault: Power, Medicine and the Body*, London: Routledge.
Atkinson, P. (1995) *Medical Talk and Medical Work*, London: Sage.

Bloor, M. and McIntosh, J. (1990) 'Surveillance and concealment: a comparison of techniques of client resistance in therapeutic communities and health visiting', in S. Cunningham-Burley and N. McKeganey (eds) *Readings in Medical Sociology*, London: Routledge.

de Swaan, A. (1990) *The Management of Normality: Critical Essays in Health and Welfare*, London: Routledge.

Ehrenreich, B. and English, D. (1974) *Complaints and Disorders: The Sexual Politics of Sickness*, London: Compendium.

Foucault, M. (1967) *Madness and Civilization: A History of Insanity in the Age of Reason*, London: Tavistock.

Foucault, M. (1975) *The Birth of the Clinic: An Archaeology of Medical Perception*, New York: Vintage Books.

Foucault, M. (1977) *Discipline and Punish: The Birth of the Prison*, London: Allen Lane.

Foucault, M. (1980) 'Body/power', in C. Gordon (ed.) *Power/Knowledge: Selected Interviews and Other Writings, 1972–1977*, New York: Pantheon.

Foucault, M. (1984a) 'Truth and power', in P. Rabinow (ed.) *The Foucault Reader*, New York: Pantheon.

Foucault, M. (1984b) 'Space, knowledge, and power', in P. Rabinow (ed.) *The Foucault Reader*, New York: Pantheon.

Foucault, M. (1986) *The Care of the Self: Volume 3 of the History of Sexuality*, New York: Pantheon.

Foucault, M. (1988) 'The political technology of individuals', in L.H. Martin, H. Gutman and P.H. Hutton (eds) *Technologies of the Self: A Seminar with Michel Foucault*, London: Tavistock.

Fox, N. (1995) 'Postmodern perspectives on care: the vigil and the gift', *Critical Social Policy*, 15, 44/5: 107–25.

Freidson, E. (1970) *Professional Dominance: The Social Structure of Medical Care*, Chicago: Aldine.

Gerhardt, U. (1989) *Ideas about Illness: An Intellectual and Political History of Medical Sociology*, New York: New York University Press.

Henriques, J., Hollway, W., Urwin, C., Venn, C. and Walkerdine, V. (1984) 'Theorizing subjectivity', in J. Henriques, W. Hollway, C. Urwin, C. Venn and V. Walkerdine, *Changing the Subject: Psychology, Social Regulation and Subjectivity*, London: Methuen.

Illich, I. (1975) *Medical Nemesis*, London: Calder and Boyars.

Lupton, D. (forthcoming) '"Your life in their hands": trust in the medical encounter', in V. James and J. Gabe (eds) *Health and the Sociology of Emotion*, Oxford: Blackwell Publishers.

May, C. (1992) 'Nursing work, nurses' knowledge, and the subjectification of the patient', *Sociology of Health & Illness*, 14, 4: 472–87.

Osborne, T. (1994) 'On anti-medicine and clinical reason', in C. Jones and R. Porter (eds) *Reassessing Foucault: Power, Medicine and the Body*, London: Routledge.

Porter, S. (1996) 'Contra-Foucault: soldiers, nurses and power', *Sociology*, 30, 1: 59–78.

Rose, N. (1994) 'Medicine, history and the present', in C. Jones and R. Porter (eds) *Reassessing Foucault: Power, Medicine and the Body*, London: Routledge.

Shilling, C. (1991) 'Educating the body: physical capital and the production of social inequalities', *Sociology*, 25, 4: 653–72.

Stein, H. (1985) *The Psychodynamics of Medical Practice: Unconscious Factors in Patient Care*, Berkeley, CA: University of California Press.

Waitzkin, H. (1984) 'The micropolitics of medicine: a contextual analysis', *International Journal of Health Services*, 14, 3: 339–78.

Zola, I. (1972) 'Medicine as an institution of social control', *Sociological Review*, 20: 487–503.

Part III

The body, the self

Chapter 6

Is health education good for you?
Re-thinking health education through the concept of bio-power

Denise Gastaldo[1]

INTRODUCTION

Traditionally, health education has been conceived as an asset within health care because it provides information and suggests alternatives to individuals, families or groups to prevent disease and promote health. From this perspective, health education seems to be a 'healthy' practice, indeed 'good for you'. This chapter intends to challenge this assumption, providing a critique of health education which employs the concept of bio-power, as developed by Michel Foucault in the first volume of his *The History of Sexuality* (1990).

Bio-power refers to the mechanisms employed to manage the population and discipline individuals. In Foucault's view, biological life is a political event: population reproduction and disease are central to economic processes and are therefore subject to political control. I employ the concept of bio-power to investigate the political dimension of health education in the arenas of health and health promotion. In this century, health has become increasingly important politically as a major point of contact between government and population. With the establishment of a net of human rights and citizenship practices, the art of government has had to develop more refined strategies in order to maintain control over the population while avoiding coercive actions. Seen from this perspective, health education can make a contribution to the exercise of bio-power because it deals with norms of healthy behaviours and promotes discipline for the achievement of good health. It is educational in nature because it promotes behaviours that should be adopted by the entire population and interferes with individual choice, providing information to foster 'healthy' lifestyles.

The central argument advanced in this chapter is that health education represents a singular contribution to the exercise of bio-power. Its involvement with prevention and health promotion, as well as its educational nature, enhance the set of power techniques that come into play in the management of individual and social bodies. The first part of this chapter discusses the concept of bio-power and how it relates to health education. The concepts of bio-politics and anatomo-politics are then explored and illustrated with data from a study on health education policies and practices in the Brazilian national health system.

BIO-POWER: THE CONCEPT

Foucault (1990: 135–9) points out that since the seventeenth century, there has been a shift in the way the population is managed, from a repressive approach to a constructive one. The sovereign's power over life was exercised by killing or abstaining from killing. However, these interventions were gradually replaced by the power to promote life. Bio-power, or power over life, constitutes power employed to control individual bodies and population. Hakosalo (1991: 9) defines bio-power as the use of mechanisms of control and coercion 'for the productivity and health of human bodies and populations', based on a view of them as 'resources and manageable objects'. Not until the eighteenth century was this kind of political rationality – concern with growth of the population and fostering of life – established (Dreyfus and Rabinow 1982: 133). Foucault (1990: 142–3) states that it was the first time in history that power concentrated on life instead of just deciding about death; biological and political existence started to interface with each other.

The body became the focus of analysis as an individual entity; it was no longer an indissociable and collective entity, like a population (Foucault 1991: 136–7). Viewing this process from a social constructionist perspective, the individual body was 'invented' at the beginning of the eighteenth century. Many power techniques have since been developed to make the body docile so that it can be 'subjected, used, transformed, and improved' (Foucault 1991: 136). Dreyfus and Rabinow (1982: 153–4) state that some form of control over the body is found in all societies. However, the employment of disciplinary power divides the body into parts and trains it, with the objective of making the parts and the whole more efficient. This happens in a subtle and continuous way, in a web of micro-powers, each including the use of space, time and everyday practices. The body has been turned into an object of knowledge. In order to govern the population, knowledge is gathered on each individual body. For the first time, the future of the society is related not only to the number of citizens and family organisation, but to the use each person makes of sex (Foucault 1990: 26). Knowledge about populations also acquired a distinct perspective in the eighteenth century. Governments recognised that dealing with populations required different strategies to those used for handling individuals. The health, illness, death and birth of populations were emerging as economic and political issues. These issues are directly related to the labour force, economic growth and distribution of wealth. In the last two centuries, population has become the target of statistical analysis and intervention measures have been designed aimed at sub-groups and the population as a whole (Foucault 1990: 146).

In order to manage the population, every individual should be reached by techniques of power. The control of the social body[2] through life demands a whole new set of strategies. For example, the practices of examining bodies, asking questions about habits and other private issues, the prescription of behaviours and drugs would not be easily accepted in health without similar experiences in other sites of social life. Foucault (1991: 28) argues that the 'body politic' relies on communication routes that construct bodies as objects of knowledge. Confession, for instance, is an important communication strategy that has been used to circulate knowledge about individual bodies. Confession, as well as the therapeutic practice of medicine, bridges the micro-physics and macro-physics of power because they link individual bodies to the social body. People are supposed to reveal their sins to their parents, to the priest, to the judge, to the doctor, to the teacher. Gordon (1991: 4–5) suggests that bio-power is the link between micro and macro; it is 'a politics concerned with subjects as members of a *population*, in which issues of individual sexual and reproductive conduct interconnect with issues of national policy and power'.

The link between the individual and the population does not mean that bio-power is a general system of domination of a group that permeates the whole social body. It is also not a set of mechanisms that guarantee control of citizens by the state (Foucault 1990: 92). Rather, bio-power is a subtle, constant and ubiquitous power over life. It is exercised through a set of power techniques, but two basic forms can be identified as the poles of this 'line of power'. In Foucault's terminology, they are the 'bio-politics of the population' and the 'anatomo-politics of the human body'. Bio-politics is the pole of bio-power that employs regulatory controls and interventions to manage the population (Foucault 1990: 139). The biological processes that are generated by the collection of individuals are directly linked to economic and social issues. For example, an epidemic may abruptly attack the labour force of a region; an increase in life expectancy implies the extension of health care and social support to elderly people. Social policy is a visible strategy to handle collective processes concerned with the life and health of the population. Other invisible power techniques, such as the expansion of the domain of the health system into private life, collaborate to gather information and to establish what is considered normal and pathological.

Anatomo-politics, at the other pole, focuses on the body as a machine (Foucault 1990: 139). Docility and usefulness are identified by Foucault as ways to integrate the body into economic and social life. In order to achieve this, the operation of disciplinary power pervades relations in families, schools, hospitals, work, etc. In the case of medicine, the effect of discipline is for the therapeutic space to become a political space. Individuality has been constructed based on symptoms, disease, or lifestyle; control over these processes is at the core of medical care (Foucault 1991: 144). The political space that health care and policy constitute is an important site for the exercise of disciplinary power. Focusing on individual bodies or on the social body, health professionals are entitled by scientific knowledge/power to examine, interview and prescribe 'healthy' lifestyles. The clinical gaze is omnipresent and acceptable because its objective is to promote health – as well as to promote a disciplinary society.

HEALTH EDUCATION AS BIO-POWER

Health education dates from the turn of the century, when the medical paradigm underwent a shift. In the nineteenth century, the predominant model was hospital medicine, concentrating on symptoms and signs that together configured a pathology (Armstrong 1995: 393). This model maintained its influence into the twentieth century, but gradually a new paradigm, surveillance medicine, has been recreating the concepts of health, illness and normality (Armstrong 1995: 394–5). Surveillance medicine moves the attention of medicine from pathological bodies to each and every member of the population. The categories of health and illness give way to the notion of risk – illness is not a problem *per se*, but a significant portion of health is redefined as an 'at-risk state' (Armstrong 1995: 400; Petersen 1996: 45–51). The borders between health and illness have also been reshaped – healthy people can become even healthier, and a person can be healthy and ill at the same time (Armstrong 1995: 400). Because ill and healthy people are 'at risk', the old tradition of teaching hygiene has proven to be insufficient, and has been transformed into the promotion of health (Armstrong 1995: 399). Health education has become part of a whole strategy to promote health for all human beings, a strategy supported by the World Health Organisation (WHO).

This shift from pathology to health for all is also noticeable in health education. Health education has been analysed in terms of the 'old' and the 'new' way of promoting health (Seymour 1984: 37). The situation is certainly more complex than a single polarity between two models. Taylor (1990: 13) reminds us that in Britain alone, there are more than seventeen taxonomies for health education. In this study, however, for the sake of clarity, health education practices that concentrate on individuals' responsibility for health and disease prevention will be called 'traditional health education'. Those practices that focus on empowering people to control their own health will be called 'radical health education'. Health education was developed under the influence of theories of disease prevention and health as a personal responsibility (Seedhouse 1986: 82; Griffiths and Adams 1991: 221). Traditional health education relates to these two concepts, as well as to reliance on professional expertise. Seedhouse (1986: 82) points out that health education still focuses on preventing diseases by providing information about food, exercise, and the risks of smoking and drinking. In the traditional approach to health education, the healthy choice is the only choice. Therefore, professionals know what the ideal choice is, and they are expected to persuade patients to lead the healthiest possible life. The possibility of a patient opting for unhealthy behaviours after some health education activity is interpreted by professionals as a failure.

The concept of radical health education figures in movements for health promotion, new public health, and healthy public policy. Radical health education focuses on empowering people to control their own health. It is also committed to combating social inequality in a broad way and promoting community participation in health issues. Within this framework, health education can be seen as a political practice that enables individuals and groups in society to organise themselves to develop actions based on their own priorities. Nevertheless, some authors (Seymour 1984: 37; Tones 1990: 2; Milio 1990: 291–7; Weare 1992: 73) have shown that many community-based projects are far from empowering communities, that healthy policies still have a long way to go before they become common practice, and that health education is still conceived in terms of campaigns designed to provide information.

Radical and traditional health education share an underlying notion of empowerment through education or subjugation through ignorance. Both are based on the understanding that human beings are liberated beings unless something oppresses them; empowering them through education is a way to remove the 'chains' of oppression – ignorance, lack of political understanding, submissive behaviours, etc. I would argue that both processes, subjugation and liberation, are acknowledged as elements of health education power relations. However, they are not the final outcome of these power/knowledge relations. What health education does construct is identity. Health education is an educational experience that gives professionals and patients/clients elements for building up representations of what is expected from 'healthy' and 'sick' people. These social roles are reinforced by a complex system of rewards and punishments. Health education is an experience of being governed from the outside and a request for self-discipline. From inside, health education is a constructive exercise of power that improves the medical gaze; through the promotion of health, it circulates everywhere in spheres that are new to bio-medicine.

The next two sections will further develop some of the points raised here, illustrated with data from a study on health education in the Brazilian national health system.

BIO-POLITICS: PARTICIPATION AND THE MANAGEMENT OF THE SOCIAL BODY[3]

In Brazil, in the early 1980s, there was a shift in the discourse of health education policy at the level of the Ministry of Health. Despite the fact that the government was a military dictatorship, a discourse of participation and empowerment through health education was beginning to be heard. A review of documents put out by the Ministry of Health from 1980 to 1992 reveals the transformation of the official discourse of health education. The 1980 Health Education Guidelines (Brasil, Ministério da Saúde 1980: 37) define health education as 'a planned activity that aims at creating conditions to produce the desired behaviour changes in relation to health'. According to the guidelines, 'the way' to carry out health education is to produce long-lasting changes in behaviour. Health education is seen as being responsible for changes, but in a very selective form. Health education means 'transferring knowledge and redefining values . . . in a pre-defined direction', but the document also suggests that the perceptions of the population should be taken into account (Brasil, Ministério da Saúde 1980: 37–8).

The proposal to promote behavioural changes 'in a pre-defined direction' raises questions about the connection between health education and bio-politics. The 'expected direction' of change is not spelled out in the document, but the implicit meaning is clearly healthier lifestyles for the population. What is healthy is what the health policy says is healthy. In other words, health education as defined in the Guidelines is intended to reinforce health patterns conceived by the government for the population. Therefore, health education policy can be understood as a strategy of governmentality through bio-politics. When health education aims to produce changes in behaviour, it becomes mainly normative. Thus, 'healthy behaviour' is presented as the norm, and all other behaviours become deviant. The principle behind the norm of behaviour is that somebody else besides the individual knows best what is appropriate or 'good for you'. This same principle, experienced in many areas of social life, is what makes governable bodies. The document further states that health education should never be coercive (Brasil, Ministério da Saúde 1980: 39). Therefore, successful health education makes people change their behaviours without feeling it as an imposition. In Foucauldian terms, the strategy suggested by the guidelines is to develop health education as a constructive power.

In 1981, when a new document was published (*Educative Action in the Basic Health Services*, Brasil, Ministério da Saúde 1981), health education policy started to make the shift from a traditional approach to promoting community participation in health activities. This policy did not focus on promoting behaviour changes. Instead, the document concentrated on the role of health centres and health professionals in promoting critical education to facilitate participation. The language and references used in the text reveal a focus on the ideas of Paulo Freire and his theory of education for liberation. The 'participatory action' proposed in this document is a recommended working method for health professionals. Community participation, presented as a partnership between professionals and users, is stressed, but the leaders of the process are the professionals. Community participation involves information about itself, contributing to the discussion of problems identified by the professionals, implementing planned actions among groups and individuals within the community, and discussing the results of plans that have been implemented (Brasil, Ministério da Saúde 1981: 10–12). Considering that this document was written while General Figueiredo's government was under military dictatorship, it appears to be quite progressive. The transition to democracy begun by that same

President may explain this tolerance of the same ideas that, in 1964, forced Paulo Freire into exile (Cowen and Gastaldo 1995: 4–5).

There is one major rupture in the discourse of the National Division of Health Education between the 1980 Guidelines and the 1981 *Educative Action in the Basic Health Services* – the way in which the community is perceived. In the first (1980) document, the community is seen as a group of individuals who would benefit from changes in their health habits, acquiring healthier lifestyles through contact with health professionals. The opinions of the community are relevant only in so far as they preclude coercive approaches to health education. In the second (1981) document, however, the community is presented as being capable of promoting health changes without the help of health professionals. The participatory method is based on the community interacting with professionals and contributing to finding solutions for problems. Although the notion of participation is not unproblematic, it represents a clear break compared with the previous document. There is some continuity in the documents. Both contain expressions (e.g. 'destitute') and references to certain kinds of social problems (e.g. garbage, water distribution, sewage treatment, etc.) that remind the reader for whom these policies are written, namely the poor, the vast majority of the Brazilian population who lack access to basic material conditions to live a decent life. Health education policy could be also analysed as a strategy for the management of some segments of the population, such as the poor.[4] However, references to such basic problems can be also understood as a commitment to those who have been oppressed throughout Brazilian history. The issue of participation is a double-edged sword: it can mean both empowerment and control. The shift from behavioural changes to 'participation' represents a new approach to the exercise of bio-politics. Rather than prescriptive norms of conduct, 'normality' should be constructed in a participatory way. The process of normalisation occurs through the creation of norms and, instead of concentrating on professionals' views, in a participatory approach the users themselves create norms and make comparisons based on these norms.

In 1982, a third document on health education was published (*Participatory Action: Methodology*, Brasil, Ministério da Saúde 1982a: 21–5). This document describes the traditional practice of health education as a combination of authoritarian-patronising methods and objectives that failed. The proposed educative action is based on the notion of a dialogue of equals – community and professionals. Respect for popular knowledge needs to be reconstructed among community and professionals, and both need to develop their critical consciousness

(Brasil, Ministério da Saúde 1982a: 10–11). Subsequent documents published in 1982, 1983 and 1984[5] continued to address the issue of health education as a strategy for participation in health. They reflected progress in terms of the discourse of participation and empowerment of users, while at the same time they helped to reshape views on the management of the population. The participatory approach respects the ideas of the group and individuals involved in health education activities. Content and methods are not imposed, and participation is expected to permeate the entire process. This constructive approach gives each individual the basic prescriptive principles of health education adapted to his or her situation. The strategy of user and professional working together to decide on health education makes the user jointly responsible for the process. A set of reactions to the prescriptive method can thus be avoided by participation.

In 1989, new guidelines were published. The document, *Health Education – Guidelines* (Brasil, Ministério da Saúde 1989: 6), addressed the daily educational practice of health professionals at all levels. The assumptions of the new guidelines do not differ substantially from assumptions made in previous documents. Once more, participation is the key concept in health education (Brasil, Ministério da Saúde 1989: 9–10). The guidelines strongly support a participatory methodology. It is participatory because health education is expected to be transformed and recreated by both professionals and community in the process of policy implementation and evaluation. In terms of bio-politics, this means that the discourse of health education has moved from repressive strategies – such as talks, demands regarding hygiene and compulsory healthy habits – to consolidating constructive tactics, such as group activities and construction of common knowledge between professionals and patients. It is worth noticing that the changes in the discourse do not necessarily relate to new practices at the health centre level.

In 1992, a new document was issued (*Education for Participation in Health*, Brasil, Ministério da Saúde 1992). The foreword outlines a 'new approach' to health education, centred on social participation, with a pedagogic model that emphasises an exchange and integration of 'knowledges' as a means to a better quality of life. Looking back to the documents produced by the National Division of Health Education in the early 1980s, there is not a huge difference between the 'new' approach described and the previous proposal of the Director of the National Division to explore alternatives based on the concepts of democratisation of health knowledge, community participation and expansion of health services (Brasil, Ministério da Saúde 1992: 1).

This brief analysis of health education policy demonstrates the thematic continuity in the discourse that federal health education policies have been circulating in the 1980s and 1990s: the issue of participation. The meaning of the term 'participation' varies from policy to policy, but from 1982 on, health education is seen as a 'method' for transforming power relations at the grassroots level. Health education is related to social science in the same way as mainstream health promotion theory at an international level, a broad trend that can also be observed in Brazil. The emphasis on participation should be seen not only as a reflection of the re-establishment of democracy in Brazil in the 1980s, but also as part of an international network in which agencies like the WHO and UNICEF disseminate trends in the health arena that deserve recognition from countries linked to the network.

An analysis of the content of these health education policies reveals that they do not concentrate on health education itself – methods, resources or topics. Instead, they propose a methodology of participation that is primarily related to the social sciences. Hewitt (1991: 243) argues that the human sciences were brought into administration and management to differentiate bodies, and to compare and classify houses, behaviours and wages. The social sciences introduced all these aspects of life into health policy. Previously, they were not considered to be part of health. The contribution this makes is to place individual bodies at the centre of the actions of professionals, who are able, thanks to the contributions of the social sciences, to judge, compare and standardise.

Looking at the discourse of health education policy on participation, social policy can be seen as a tool for the 'circulation of power' or as 'capillaries in the social body' (Hewitt 1991: 230–1), since policy can promote constructive power relations in the management of the social body. However, the capillary metaphor may create a false image of the way social policy relates to bio-politics. The idea of circulation of power assumes that social policy achieves implementation, and that there is coherent articulation between various levels of government and those in charge of policy implementation. Some examples of the policy process illustrate the complexity of the cluster of power relations that occur in the exercise of bio-politics. What emerges from an examination of implementation of federal health education policy is the lack of concrete achievement of such policies (Gastaldo 1996: 116–19, 137–9). Perhaps we should use the terminology of Easton (quoted in Ham 1992: 94–5) to describe Brazilian health education policy: the policy of inaction. The Brazilian national health system traditionally discriminated against part of the population (those not formally engaged in the workforce); policies failed to establish objectives or a schedule for implementation at the national level; no demands were made on state or municipal governments in terms of implementation. In this context, how could the discourse of participation become a social practice at the grassroots level? The path to transformation chosen by the National Division of Health Education was nothing more than 'telling' health centres to adopt participatory practices.

According to information provided by health centres in Rio Grande do Sul (a Brazilian state) in 1993, community participation is conceived in a variety of ways. The most frequent pattern is not to have any form of community participation in health centres (Gastaldo 1996: 179–82). Among those who mentioned participation, there are references to the community helping with vaccination campaigns or writing complaints and requests to put in the 'suggestion box'. The presence of a community representative (either informally chosen or formally elected) at the health centre is a rare occurrence.

Looking at policy formulation at various levels of government, the lack of articulation between health education policies *per se* and health policies in general leads one to question how power is circulated through social policy (Gastaldo 1996: 140–68). Observation of implementation strategies at the health centres raises the same issue. In the selection of priorities, the profession and specialism of the head of the health centre may be influential; the number of professionals working there and their views on the community may also impede policy implementation (Gastaldo 1996: 188–95).

What the above examples illustrate is that social policy is not a single stream of power from the federal to the local level. The process of promoting knowledge and norms occurs within a web of micro-powers of forms of control and resistance. Even when health education policy is articulated at all levels of government and delivers the central government discourse to health centres, the discourse will face resistance there and will be reconstructed. Micro-politics at the grassroots level can be a powerful source of resistance. In the Brazilian context, 'understandings' of and traditions in health education are as important for health centres as policies sent to them by the government (Gastaldo 1996: 116).

Health education policy may therefore appear not to be an efficient strategy for the circulation of power. However, federal health education policy has been written down and distributed as a form of circulating ideas. The discourse of participation is the predominant discourse today. Perhaps it was accepted in the first place because it relates to the international discourse of health promotion, some policy-makers were committed to transformative principles, and it was convenient for a government making the transition to democracy. Nevertheless, that discourse later became quite influential in the reform of the national health system and was turned into practice in some health institutions (Gastaldo 1996: 94–102, 246–55).

The analysis of the policy process challenges the simplistic notion that the government can manage the social body through social policy or that social policy is a single and coherent strategy of power. The concept of bio-politics must be understood according to Foucault's general framework of power relations (1990: 94): 'power is exercised from innumerable points, in the interplay of nonegalitarian and mobile relations. . . . there is no binary and all-encompassing opposition between rulers and ruled at the root of power relations'. In fact, traditional and radical approaches are extreme forms of the exercise of power present at all levels of the policy process; these approaches occur in parallel with discourses and practices of different intensity. What happens in the contact between the population and the national health system in terms of health education activities is far more complex than what is stated in the official policy.

ANATOMO-POLITICS: LEARNING TO BE A HEALTHY CITIZEN

The concept of anatomo-politics is useful in examining the user's experience of this contact. According to Foucault, anatomo-politics involves the docilisation of individual bodies.

> [it is] . . . centered on the body as a machine: its disciplining, the optimization of its capabilities, the extortion of its forces, the parallel increase of its usefulness and its docility, its integration into systems of efficient and economic controls, all this was ensured by the procedures of power that characterized the *disciplines*: an *anatomo-politics of the human body*.
>
> (Foucault 1990: 139)

Anatomo-politics became part of daily life, an invisible power, with no exteriority, but tangled in the relations of knowledge, surveillance, and so on that discipline bodies. Ewald (1992: 169–75) argues that discipline was transformed from a negative form – such as blocking the poor and insane in society – to a mechanism that targets bodies in order to train them. Ewald points out that:

> Disciplines are no longer the prerogative of certain institutions. . . . Disciplines become ubiquitous and liberated, no longer addressing only someone who is to be punished . . . they are placed at the service of the good, the good of all, of all socially useful production. Disciplines are addressed to all people, without distinction.
>
> (Ewald 1992: 169–70)

Foucault (1991: 170) states that 'discipline "makes" individuals'; individuals are objects, and instruments of this specific technique of power. The process of disciplining bodies is also accomplished through the meticulous regulation of 'the smallest fragments of life' (Foucault 1991: 140). For users of the national health system, there are rules and norms for gaining access to every small procedure they request. This experience of discipline is reinforced by mechanisms for minor punishment or reward, based on the individual 'performances' of the users.

Gaining access to the services of the Brazilian national health system involves observing a set of rules. The rules encompass surveillance, control of space, and codes of behaviour, from patients in the queue and health professionals in charge of the process. The health centre opens at 7 a.m. and there are ten *fichas* (tokens for consultation) for the paediatrician, which will be distributed to the first to arrive in the queue. It is not possible to obtain a token by simply making a telephone call or writing a letter. Someone must be physically present to get the token. Patients are very concerned that queuing procedures are properly observed. Before a health centre has opened, patients organise the queue according to the number of tokens for each specialism and tell those who exceed the number of tokens available that they have little chance of obtaining a consultation. Queuing is part of everyday life for users of the national health system. During the fieldwork upon which this chapter is based, one patient was observed arriving, saying 'Good morning', then asking: 'Who is the last one in the queue?' The patient joined the end of the queue in silence to have a bandage changed.

There is no way to use the national health system without queuing up for hours. Because it is a compulsory experience, the 'outcomes' of this practice can be shocking. Before the health centre opens, people stand outside the building. Despite the fact that on winter nights the temperature may be as low as 0–5°C, women queue for hours with all their children. Because some women are single parents or their partners start work very early, they have no other alternative than to take the whole family to the health centre and queue up. Each adult is limited to one consultation per specialist, so a mother with two sick children needs to take another adult along with her. If both children have the same disease, she may be able to persuade the person at the reception desk to give her two consultations, but two or three different consultations will make things very difficult for her. In the health centres observed, the staff would try to accommodate a consultation for a second child, but a third would mean yet another night in the queue.

These observations on access show that the national health system establishes a particular relationship with users. The user does not exist for the system unless the person is physically present. The body has to be present for the existence of the person to be acknowledged and patient status to be given as a reward. This prerequisite creates the opportunity to make the national health system an experience of disciplining bodies. Foucault mentions the training of every part of the body to achieve discipline. In the national health system, from childhood, the individual body stands for hours in a queue and copes with cold weather, rain and sleep deprivation. The body is kept under surveillance, and helps keep control over other bodies.

After obtaining a token and having a consultation, some patients will be referred to health education activities. Two experiences of focus groups observed during fieldwork are described below to illustrate the potential of health education for subjugation and empowerment. One of the observed focus groups for pregnant women was presented to the patients as an opportunity to talk, resolve doubts and discuss issues of interest to the participants. There was no specific content to be taught. The choice of topics was up to the patients. Compared to other health education groups, this approach is more patient-centred. The dynamic of the group was structured by patients asking questions and professionals answering them. Professionals made an effort to listen to patients' opinions and experiences from previous pregnancies. However, any technical aspect raised (for example, whether or not a pregnant woman should take aspirin, whether or not there is any problem with going to the dentist) was presented directly to the doctor in the group. The criterion of normality was in his hands.

The question of what is normal and what is not was raised five times during the one-hour session. Here is a typical exchange:

Patient	Sometimes I sleep and a white substance, it's a milk, something very sticky, spreads in my clothes. I am not sure if this is normal.
Doctor	It is normal. But it is also normal for it not to happen.

The two main features of these meetings for pregnant women were the professionals', especially the doctors', attempt to control the 'correct' or final answer and reinforce the importance of the professional–patient relationship. Here are some more exchanges from the same meeting:

Doctor	Theoretically, all doctors know which drugs you can take or not. So, if the doctor recommends a medication you can take it with confidence. . . . If the baby sucks and the mother goes to the paediatrician periodically, and the baby is putting on weight, for sure the quantity and quality of milk the baby is receiving is sufficient . . . if he doesn't put weight on properly, the paediatrician will detect that. If the person needs an X-ray, there is a lead jacket that protects the tummy from radiation, and the doctor will always calculate the risk and the benefit.

In their answers to the group, the doctors were reassuring about the trust the patient should have in any doctor. The healthy pregnant citizen is one who participates and looks for information, but is also a docile body. Health information should be disseminated among patients, and patients have the power to choose the issues they want to discuss, but scientific knowledge entitles professionals to control the boundaries of normality and thus to construct 'normal' bodies.

Patients in the hypertension group come in to have their blood pressure checked and get their medication. The contact with the doctor is also used for quick *ad hoc* consultations. What is particular to this group is the medicalisation of daily life and the extension of the concept of health through the notion of risk. In a meeting coordinated by a nurse, patients were discussing their condition. The issues discussed included food, physical activities, work, television programs, relatives and shopping. At the next meeting, the same group was coordinated by the doctor, who brought up the issue of conditions in the health centre. During the discussion, patients revealed some of the codes of conduct that are part of the group.

Doctor	Here in the group we are all the same, everybody has the right to speak. Of course, there are personal differences; Mrs. Silva, for instance, rarely speaks. We can see that she is a quiet person.
Patient 1	She doesn't have the right to talk because she comes late (laughter).
Patient 2	But today she came early.
Doctor	Yes, today she came early. It is important to have the right but also to consider yourself equal to others . . .
Patient 3	We should talk when we know, but when we don't know, we should stay quiet.

The meeting was very political; patients decided to write a letter and make an appointment with the mayor of the city to request better material conditions for the health centre and other improvements. Negotiations about who should take responsibility for getting the process started were initiated, as usual, by the doctor.

Patient 1	So why don't you write a letter, doctor?
Doctor	Why me? The group should do it.
(Comments)	
Doctor	How can we do it? To whom should we send the letter?
Patient 2	To the mayor, of course.
Doctor	Does everybody agree?
(All patients agree.)	
Patient 1	Wait a minute, who will write the letter?
Patient 3	I volunteer to walk and deliver the letter (laughter).
Patient 4	. . . We want the health centre working day and night.

The experience of writing a letter, organising the group, and meeting the mayor to present a request is seen here as radical health education to patients suffering of hypertension. The patients were worried about being 'humble' people and not being received by the mayor, and about writing a letter in good Portuguese. This meeting promoted the empowerment of the users, encouraging community organisation. At the same time, this experience involves the medicalisation of life – promotion of health through access to medical care.

A feature of this group was that complaints about the difficulties of being a user of the national health system were not ignored, but discussed in the group. Health education, in this case, was intended to share solutions and resist forms of control over individual and collective bodies identified by the patients. The important point, however, is that this approach does not eliminate the disciplinary experience of being a user of the national health system and the intrinsic mechanisms of power that pervade health education activities: surveillance of the community, self-discipline as a positive outcome of health education practice, and the production of healthy citizens who disseminate the domain of health into life in general.

Health education activities can promote a critical position on the part of the community, promoting an understanding of health as a political and socio-economic experience. The organisation of groups within the community, an increased understanding of the body and body processes, and making room for political action within the health centre are among the results of a radical approach to health education. The construction of the 'healthy citizen' occurs in this milieu, and what is added to the process is the context of health. The clinical gaze over the community is carried out not only by health professionals, but by everyone involved in health education activities; they bring the community into the health centre, carrying with them the concepts of a 'regime of total health'. Health thus becomes synonymous with life.

IS HEALTH EDUCATION GOOD FOR YOU?

It is 'plain common sense' to say that health education 'is good for you'. In a country like Brazil, where educational resources are limited, being in contact with health professionals and learning about one's own body and the health of one's family is clearly a good opportunity. Seen from this perspective, health education is indeed a 'healthy' practice, a 'good thing'.

A more detailed analysis of this issue, however, reveals that health education covers a large range of practices, from 'good' to 'bad', from 'healthy' to 'unhealthy', from empowerment to subjugation, and from liberation to docilisation. Health education is empowerment because the information provided to patients helps them to make informed choices. Based on the knowledge acquired and their own previous knowledge, patients can make decisions about their health, taking into account scientific, social and personal factors. This gives them an opportunity to exercise autonomy and self-government. The political dimension of health education also makes it a site for involvement in the micro-politics of the community, as well as a transmission belt for requests to the different levels of government.

Health education is also subjugation. Many health education practices involve the imposition of 'truths' about health, in which the patient loses control of her or his own body. Instead of choice, the patient experiences the government of her or his body or family from outside. Health education can also mean control because it extends the clinical gaze over the population. Health education covers most of the issues related to life, and is put into practice by a network of professionals, from social workers to psychologists. This double view of health education is based upon the idea that total autonomy and liberation are not possible for any human being. According to Foucault's theory, no educational process can only liberate because at the same time it disciplines bodies. Therefore, health education is seen here as both empowerment and subjugation.

Health education is normally taken for granted as being a good practice. Practices and policies suggest that health education has not been challenged in its constituent elements (e.g. confession, self-discipline, etc.), but has been reformed or transformed in its general strategies of approach – from traditional practices to participatory practices. As bio-politics, health education policies have been disseminating discourses of participation and empowerment. This means that the health system is turning from repressive approaches to constructive approaches to manage the population. As anatomo-politics, health education is exercised in the promotion of health. Whether healthy or sick, the 'healthy citizen' keeps in touch with the national health system because health education activities are for all, preventing disease and promoting health. Therefore, health education, through its capacity of expanding the limits of health practice into the healthy community, is an exercise of power over life.

Returning to our initial question, 'Is health education good for you?', the answer is: it may well be. However, health education certainly contributes to the management of social and individual bodies.

NOTES

1 I would like to thank the Editors of this volume, as well as Eva Gamarnikow, Bob Cowen, Michel Perreault, Ernesto Jaramillo and Flavio Kapczinski, for their critical comments.
2 The expressions 'social body' and 'collective body' are not figurative. Barret-Kriegel (1992: 194) comments that the term 'body' represents a 'complex and multiple materiality' and that talking about the social body emphasises its physical element.
3 The information provided in the next two sections was collected during fieldwork in Brazil in 1993. The methodology of the research is described in Gastaldo (1996: 50–70).

4 The relationship between the national health system and the government of the poor is further developed in Gastaldo (1996: 95–17).

5 Documents published during that period: *Participatory Action: Evaluating Experiences* (1982b); *Participatory Action: Human Resources Education* (1982c); *Participatory Action: Production of Educational Materials* (1983); *Participatory Action: Perspectives on Health Education Practice* (1984).

BIBLIOGRAPHY

Armstrong, D. (1995) 'The rise of surveillance medicine', *Sociology of Health & Illness*, 17, 3: 393–404.

Barret-Kriegel, B. (1992) 'Michel Foucault and the police state', in T.J. Armstrong (ed. and trans.) *Michel Foucault, Philosopher: International Conference*, London: Routledge.

Beattie, A. (1991) 'Knowledge and control in health promotion: a test case for social policy and social theory', in J. Gabe, M. Calnan and M. Bury (eds) *The Sociology of the Health Service*, London: Routledge.

Brasil, Ministério da Saúde (1980) *Educação em saúde nas unidades federadas* [Health education in the federation unities], Brasília: Ministério da Saúde.

Brasil, Ministério da Saúde (1981) *Ação educativa nos serviços básicos de saúde* [Educative action in the basic health services], Brasília: Ministério da Saúde.

Brasil, Ministério da Saúde (1982a) *Ação participativa: metodologia* [Participatory action: methodology], Brasília: Ministério da Saúde.

Brasil, Ministério da Saúde (1982b) *Ação participativa: avaliação de experiências* [Participatory action: evaluating experiences], Brasília: Ministério da Saúde.

Brasil, Ministério da Saúde (1982c) *Ação participativa: capacitação de pessoal* [Participatory action: human resources education], Brasília: Ministério da Saúde.

Brasil, Ministério da Saúde (1983) *Ação participativa: produção de materiais instrucionais* [Participatory action: production of educational materials], Brasília: Ministério da Saúde.

Brasil, Ministério da Saúde (1984) *Ação participativa: perspectivas de atuação dos educadores de saúde pública* [Participatory action: perspectives on health education practice], Brasília: Ministério da Saúde.

Brasil, Ministério da Saúde (1989) *Educação em saúde – diretrizes* [Health education – guidelines], Brasília: Ministério da Saúde.

Brasil, Ministério da Saúde (1992) *Educação para a participação em saúde* [Education for participation in health], Brasília: Ministério da Saúde.

Bunton, R. (1992) 'Health promotion as social policy', in R. Bunton and G. Macdonald *Health Promotion – Disciplines and Diversity*, London: Routledge.

Canguilhem, G. (1989) *The Normal and Pathological*, New York: Zone Books.

Caplan, R. and Holland, R. (1990) 'Rethinking health education theory', *Health Education Journal*, 49, 1: 10–12.

Catford, J. and Nutbeam, D. (1984) 'Towards the definition of health education and health promotion', *Health Education Journal*, 43, 2–3: 38.

Codd, J. (1988) 'The construction and deconstruction of educational policy documents', *Journal of Education Policy*, 3, 3: 235–47.

Cowen, M.F. and Gastaldo, D. (1995) *Paulo Freire at the Institute*, London: Institute of Education.

Crawford, R. (1980) 'Healthism and the medicalisation of everyday life', *International Journal of Health Services*, 10, 3: 365–88.

Dean, M. (1992) 'A genealogy of the government of poverty', *Economy and Society*, 21, 3: 215–51.

Donnelly, M. (1992) 'On Foucault's uses of the notion "biopower"', in T.J. Armstrong (ed. and trans.) *Michel Foucault, Philosopher: International Conference*, London: Routledge.

Dreyfus, H. and Rabinow, P. (1982) *Michel Foucault – Beyond Structuralism and Hermeneutics*, Brighton: Harvester Press.

Ewald, F. (1992) 'A power without exterior', in T.J. Armstrong (ed. and trans.) *Michel Foucault, Philosopher: International Conference*, London: Routledge.

Foucault, M. (1970) *The Order of Things – An Archaeology of the Human Sciences*, New York: Random House.

Foucault, M. (1976) 'Governmentality', *Ideology and Consciousness*, 6: 5–21.

Foucault, M. (1990) *The History of Sexuality*, Volume I: *An Introduction*, London: Penguin.

Foucault, M. (1991) *Discipline and Punish – The Birth of the Prison*, London: Penguin.

Gastaldo, D. (1996) 'Is health education good for you? The social construction of health education in the Brazilian national health system', PhD thesis, University of London.

Gordon, C. (1991) 'Governmental rationality: an introduction', in G. Burchell, C. Gordon and P. Miller (eds) *The Foucault Effect: Studies in Governmental Rationality*, Hemel Hempstead: Harvester Wheatsheaf.

Griffiths, J. and Adams, L. (1991) 'The new health promotion', in P. Draper (ed.) *Health through Public Policy*, London: Grenn Print.

Hakosalo, H. (1991) *Bio-power and Pathology*, Oulu: University of Oulu Press.

Ham, C. (1992) *Health Policy in Britain*, 3rd edn, London: Macmillan.

Hewitt, M. (1991) 'Bio-politics and social policy: Foucault's account of welfare', in M. Featherstone, M. Hepworth and B. Turner (eds) *The Body – Social Process and Cultural Theory*, London: Sage.

Lupton, D. (1995) *The Imperative of Health – Public Health and the Regulated Body*, London: Sage.

Milio, N. (1990) 'Healthy cities: the new public health and supportive research', *Health Promotion International*, 5, 4: 291–7.

Pederson, A., Edwards, R., Marshall, V., Allison, K. and Kelner, M. (1989) *Coordinating Healthy Public Policy – An Analytic Literature Review and Bibliography*, Toronto: Minister of National Health and Welfare.

Petersen, A. (1996) 'Risk and the regulated self: the discourse of health promotion as politics of uncertainty', *Australian & New Zealand Journal of Sociology*, 32, 1: 44–57.

Rodmell, S. and Watt, A. (eds) (1986) *The Politics of Health Education*, London: Routledge.

Seedhouse, D. (1986) *Health – The Foundations for Achievement*, Chichester: John Wiley and Sons.

Seymour, H. (1984) 'Health education versus health promotion – a practitioner's view', *Health Education Journal*, 43, 2–3: 37–8.

Taylor, V. (1990) 'Health education – a theoretical mapping', *Health Education Journal*, 49, 1: 13–14.

Tones, K. (1990) 'Why theorise? Ideology in health education', *Health Education Journal*, 49, 1: 2–6.

Weare, K. (1992) 'The contribution of education to health promotion', in R. Bunton and G. Macdonald (eds) *Health Promotion – Disciplines and Diversity*, London: Routledge.

Chapter 7

Bodies at risk
Sex, surveillance and hormone replacement therapy

Jennifer Harding

BACKGROUND

Hormone replacement therapy (HRT) has attracted public attention as a technology claimed to slow down the natural degeneration and 'de-feminisation' of the ageing female body. It is a medically prescribed treatment which, in medical terms, is designed to remedy the pathological effects of oestrogen deficiency occurring at, and defining, the onset of menopause and subsequent postmenopause. HRT, it is claimed, is capable of preventing physical and mental disease, loss of libido and sexual attractiveness resulting from reduced levels of natural oestrogen in older women's bodies (Gorman and Whitehead 1989). Since oestrogen is commonly represented as the stereotypical female sex hormone and the biological basis of femininity (Oudshoum 1994; Harding 1996), the widespread promotion of HRT has come to signal, in a broader cultural context, an attempt to maintain and reinforce sexual difference.

Female sex hormones, since early this century, have been significant objects of bio-medical research, resulting in a variety of clinical applications. Sex hormones, especially female sex hormones, have achieved a more global and popular significance, beyond medical discourse, as all-powerful masters of mood, sexuality, appearance and behaviour (Harding 1993). Recently, medical experts have claimed that the prescription of HRT should be routine and long term on the grounds that oestrogen replacement affords postmenopausal women protection against the 'risks' of developing serious debilitating and potentially fatal diseases like cardiovascular disease and osteoporosis (Law *et al.* 1991; Stampfer *et al.* 1991; MacLennan 1992; Wren 1992). This claim has led medical experts to advise women to seek prolonged treatment for long-term disease and transient symptoms from menopause until death (Goldman and Tosteson 1991; *The Lancet* 1991; MacLennan 1991; Moon 1991). One consequence of such advice is that huge new markets of consumers requiring both pharmaceuticals and screening services (to detect possible adverse effects accompanying this treatment) are potentially opened up. Another consequence is that significant areas of women's bodily experiences are progressively subjected to techniques of medical surveillance.

Medical claims that menopause constitutes a disease requiring treatment and that HRT may prevent growing decrepitude and sexual redundancy have been widely promulgated through various media channels. However, HRT has not met with unbridled enthusiasm. Since its first vigorous promotion in the 1960s, HRT has been considered controversial and its efficacy and *safety* have been consistently challenged.[1] Against the therapeutic claims made for HRT, it has been argued that the effectiveness of HRT as a prophylactic has not been adequately proven (Klein 1992; Worcester and Whately 1992).[2] It has also been argued that use of HRT may be associated with an increased incidence of other diseases like breast and endometrial cancers (Coney 1991) and that, therefore, the risks of taking HRT may exceed the risks of not taking it (Coney 1991). Further, it is claimed that it is sexist to assume, as Robert Wilson (1966) first did, that menopause results in de-feminisation unless treated with synthetic hormones (Greer 1991; Vines 1993). These arguments have been made largely by feminists writing on women's health issues who have attributed the successful deployment of HRT to the medicalisation of the menopause (thereby defining a normal life process as a disease needing treatment) and the commercial exploitation of fear within a contemporary Western cultural matrix of sexism and ageism (Coney 1991; Klein 1992; Worcester and Whately 1992). Feminists have argued that, as an alternative and preferable means to preventing disease, women should be better informed about 'the normal healthy workings' of their bodies and choices and encouraged to adopt healthy lifestyles (Worcester and Whately 1992).

Regardless of the actual number of women who swallow, affix or apply it, the deployment of HRT defines menopause as a nodal point in women's lives and constitutes *all* women as a coherent potential treatment group based on reproductive processes in common. It marks postmenopause as a uniform time of ageing, stretching between menopause and death, differentiated from pre-menopause by specific symptoms and disease (Harding 1993). Importantly, it emphasises the ideas that hormones are measurable and adjustable chemical indicators of sex (Harding 1993; Oudshoorn 1994) and that sex hormones are responsible for distinguishing female from male, disease from health, infertile from fertile, desired from desiring (Harding 1993).

The deployment of HRT in response to medically diagnosed oestrogen deficiency underlines the idea that there is something basically missing in the female body. Further, since the idea still lingers, from early twentieth-century medical discourse, that hormones are chemical messengers whose function is to transmit the appropriate details of femininity and masculinity (Long Hall 1973; Harding 1993; Oudshoorn 1994), the semantics of oestrogen deficit and replacement place femininity in question. Femininity is rendered precarious, provisional and in need of reinforcement. Indeed, HRT is fast becoming a significant 'technology of power' (Foucault 1979: 30, 1981: 12) thanks to medical claims that it (HRT) is capable of remedying an ever-growing list of defects attributable to oestrogen deficiency and seen as undermining femininity (Harding 1993).

Discourse on HRT centres on a range of symptoms and diseases (related to menopause and postmenopause) which operate as 'secondary sex characteristics' and expressions of an original female body. In this way, discourse on HRT participates in producing and sexing the natural body. HRT marks a crossroads in contemporary discourse on sex, which is focused almost exclusively on the postmenopausal woman.

HRT has become the focus of vigorous and pervasive debate to the extent that Renate Klein argues that for 'most women' now facing middle age, the question of whether or not to take HRT is becoming one of 'paramount importance' (Klein 1992: 25). Debate is largely focused on the risks of using or not using HRT. Different experts and commentators, medical and feminist, have endeavoured to establish a convincing computation of the relative risks and benefits of this treatment. Each group seeks to inform women of their 'options'. All actively contribute to an 'epidemic of signification' (Treichler 1987) and information-generation which constitutes as its target a subject, the postmenopausal woman, whose existence is becoming ever more ambiguous as it hovers on the borders of normality/pathology and celebration/erasure. Each commentator encourages the postmenopausal woman to engage in practices of self-surveillance and presumes that she is willing to do so. Each presumes that health is a paramount cultural value and an ideal readily pursued by all women.

FOUCAULT AND HRT

An analysis of HRT in terms of its potential benefits and/or risks, whether from a medical or an alternative perspective (for example, feminist discourse on women's health), does not fully explore the possible significances of this technology. Indeed, debate about the pros and cons limits what might be said about HRT. Such debate, in foregrounding concerns about protecting women from risks of disease, tends to represent as unproblematic the categories *women* and *risk*. Postmenopausal women are represented as a generic category and as sharing a singular political positioning in relation to medical practitioners. Risk is represented as a self-evident danger to be avoided.

An alternative perspective views HRT as a contemporary 'technology of power', and, following Foucault, centres on the mobility of discourse, including its functions in the production of power relations and subjectivity, and the multiplicity of sites of power and resistance. Here, I examine how medical and feminist discourses on HRT constitute the subjects of whom and to whom they speak – in this case, postmenopausal women at risk of developing disease – and how they participate in the sexing of bodies.

Relevant to this analysis are the ideas that discourses constitute social phenomena, that they are practices, and operate as fields of fluid and mobile 'relations' and 'interrelations' which produce and transmit power/knowledge, where power and knowledge directly imply one another (Foucault 1979, 1981, 1986).[3] Also relevant are the ideas that the subject who knows, the objects to be known and the modalities of knowledge are all the effects of historically specific transformations of relations of power/knowledge and are produced, transmitted and reinforced in discourse.[4] The construction of the subject of discourse within power relations is always an incomplete process (Foucault 1986; Butler 1992).

I examine what I broadly term 'medical discourse' and 'women's health discourse', without implying that either of these is a uniform discourse, or is diametrically opposed to the other or that they constitute a dominant and dominated discourse.[5] Foucault suggests that there is neither a dominant nor dominated discourse but a 'multiplicity of discursive elements that can come into play in various strategies', whereby there might exist 'different and even contradictory discourses within the same strategy' and discourses might circulate without changing form from one strategy to another (Foucault 1981: 100–2). Medical discourse and women's health discourse can be seen as key nodes of enunciation in a discursive field centring on HRT. However, they are not the only discourses on HRT, nor are they coherent and/or mutually exclusive. Each is distinguished by typical goals, strategies and points of opposition to the other.

In different ways, both medical and women's health discourses participate in the construction of a (post)menopausal woman who is in need of a detailed knowledge of the risks she faces in order to control her destiny. The construct *risk*, and the opportunities it provides for surveillance, provide common ground for medical and feminist discourses and a direct point of address, and hence access, to the individual, whereby she is constituted and positioned as a sexed subject. In the following paragraphs, I examine some key aspects of discourses on HRT to show how bodies may become sexed in discourse.

THE POSTMENOPAUSAL WOMAN

In addressing 'women' as 'a univocal positioning' (Butler 1990a), all discourses on HRT define the usual characteristics of, and conditions of belonging to, this generic category of subjects. Medical and women's health discourses on HRT address a postmenopausal woman who possesses a body circumscribed by its reproductive capacity and is at risk of developing disease. She is problematised at the level of what she 'chooses' to do about it (Harding 1993).

The discursively constructed postmenopausal woman is a corporeal terrain, normal and pathological, demarcated by the clean intersection of the discrete and finite categories age and sex. In medical discourse, the body of the postmenopausal woman is the site of a sex-linked disease of endocrine deficiency producing both short-term symptoms and long-term disease and occasioning medical intervention, including treatment and surveillance, for *all* women from menopause until death (Gorman and Whitehead 1989; Goldman and Tosteson 1991; *The Lancet* 1991; MacLennan 1991; Moon 1991). The medically constructed postmenopausal woman faces up to the adverse effects of oestrogen deficiency out of fear and ignorance.

It has been claimed that coronary heart disease ranks as 'number one in the causes of major disability in later life' (MacLennan 1991) and 'the most common cause of death in women' (Goldman and Tosteson 1991: 800); osteoporosis constitutes 'a major cause of morbidity in women' (Goldman and Tosteson 1991: 800); and menopausal symptomatology is 'a leading cause of discomfort in women' (Goldman and Tosteson 1991: 800). However, it is also acknowledged that HRT is not widely used, at least in the UK. Low usage of HRT is attributed to resistance by women and clinicians based on misconceptions of adverse effects, mainly fear of cancer and withdrawal bleeding and women's failure to comply with treatments.[6] Authors of medical texts use risk–benefit calculations to dismiss perceived fears of 'the presumed adverse effects' of HRT (*The Lancet* 1991: 917), without considering whether, and how, statistical computations make sense to differently positioned women. The antidote to low usage, some authors suggest, lies in tailoring and individualising treatment to minimise unwanted effects, like reducing the frequency of withdrawal bleeding (*The Lancet* 1991: 918; MacLennan 1991: 43).[7] Medical authors also argue that not all women will benefit equally from long-term use of HRT. Rather, 'the challenge for the 1990s is to identify those women who would benefit most and to ensure that they receive adequate therapy' (*The Lancet* 1991: 918). However, few women are likely to be consistently excluded, since the idea that 'all women should be assessed at the menopause and counselled about their options' (MacLennan 1991: 44) assumes that medical consultation is normal for menopausal women. At the same time, this process of normalisation relies upon and reinforces a systematic exclusion of women who do not have access to this form of health care or who are constructed as unlikely to benefit from treatment – for example, poor and black women.[8]

In women's health discourse, the body of the postmenopausal woman is constituted as the site of 'normal' physiological processes (like the end of her reproductive life) not typically requiring treatment, but subjected to the colonising strategies of medicalisation and commercialisation (National Women's Health Network 1989; Coney 1991; Klein 1992; Worcester and Whately 1992). Several feminist authors argue that the medicalisation of the menopause has been made possible and fuelled by its potential to generate lucrative markets for (commercially run) services providing pharmaceuticals, tests and investigations (Coney 1991; Greer 1991; Klein 1992; Worcester and Whately 1992). These texts produce a postmenopausal woman who is at risk of exploitation as her real needs are subordinated to the interests of medical career-making and commercial profit. She is at risk of the adverse health effects of HRT through lack of information and bombardment with misinformation about the true effects of HRT, which defines her as sick and therefore disempowers her, sending her on 'an endless quest for the Holy Grail of youth and perfect health' (Coney 1991: 20). According to Sandra Coney, the medicalisation of the menopause means that the mid-life woman is caught in a bind, contemplating the consequences of both accepting and refusing treatment and accompanying investigations (Coney 1991: 16). Whilst women may feel 'healthy and fit in their natural state' there is always 'a niggling doubt, a sneaking suspicion that some vile, sinister disease process is all the while surreptitiously invading some body part, rendering bones in danger of imminent collapse, breasts about to erupt with mountainous lumps' (Coney 1991: 16).

Feminist health writers call for better research and availability to women of relevant information about 'true' (adverse as well as remedial) effects of using HRT, alternative non-pharmaceutical approaches to symptom relief and disease prevention (for example, healthy lifestyles) and knowledge about the 'normal healthy workings' of their bodies (Coney 1991; Greer 1991; Klein 1992; Worcester and Whately 1992). Such information enables women to 'make informed choices' about their health care options, to wrestle control away from medical practitioners and become empowered (Worcester and Whately 1992: 23). In the tradition of analyses generated by, and characterising, a 'women's health movement', these statements constitute a cogent challenge to medical discursive practices. They have been politically significant in assisting many women to articulate consumer demands and participate actively in questioning and defining health care options. However, they tend to construct the postmenopausal woman as a generic entity occupying one of two possible subject positions: either sick, misinformed, over-dependent on medications and disempowered; or well, informed, engaging in non-medical and self-help practices and empowered. Women progress along an axis of disempowerment/ empowerment as they gain access to knowledge. This conceptualisation obscures the ways in which women are differently placed in relation to each other, with different capacities to challenge prevailing relations of power. This discursive strategy also produces the postmenopausal woman as a passive recipient of knowledge.

In the above scenario, the female body is typically positioned as a site of oppression and liberation based on acquisition of knowledge of it. Lack of freedom and heteronomy are produced as causes of 'a false relation to the body' (Haug 1987: 248). Requests for unbiased and accurate information about the real risks of HRT are largely articulated in the medical idiom of risks and benefits and medical understandings of disease and physiology (detailing the 'normal', 'natural' and 'healthy' body). 'The body' therefore becomes a site for the application of knowledge generated elsewhere (Haug 1987). Furthermore, an unquestioning acceptance of the categories nominated in medical discourse implies that knowledge is a neutral and transparent instrument, which once possessed will liberate the formerly oppressed. Knowledge appears neutral because it is constructed as external to power (Haug 1987). Contrary to this, Frigga Haug argues 'If liberating forms of thought and action are to be possible, it will be necessary to transform the very concepts through which knowledge becomes accessible' (Haug 1987: 251).

Both medical and women's health discourses on HRT address a generic postmenopausal woman who needs information in order to assess the risks she faces and make informed choices about how to handle her menopause. A concentrated focus on menopause as a nodal point in all women's lives and the threshold of older womanhood eclipses consideration of health problems which may reflect the ways in which gendered positioning intersects with other political positionings determined, for example, by the unequal relations of race and class.

RISK AND RESPONSIBILITY

The medical construction of menopause as a disease of deficiency giving rise to symptoms and diseases, like hot flushes and cardiovascular disease, brings into being a population whose health is endangered in a common, though individualised, way through the concept of 'risk'. Risk implies that disease could strike the unwary and careless at any time. Medical discourse tends to assume that individuals are attuned to a 'rationalist understanding of reality' implicit in a 'discourse on risk' in which things do not happen without warning and 'unfortunate events are deemed to be both predictable and avoidable' (Lupton 1995: 79). The use of HRT, like other interventions to prevent disease, appears to constitute a strategy aimed at diminishing uncertainty. Feminist critiques of HRT also employ a discourse on risk. In both medical and women's health discourses, perceived susceptibility to risk is essential in motivating behaviour (Lupton 1995: 82) and this perception is facilitated by the supply of information (Lupton 1995: 77) about ways of preventing disease (whether dietary or pharmacological).

Medical texts advocating long-term use of HRT emphasise that fatality and debility caused by cardiovascular disease and osteoporosis are needless and articulate a public health rationale. For example, with regard to osteoporosis, it is claimed that fractures are avoidable and, therefore, suffering as a result of broken bones is needless. It is asserted that fractures are financially costly, drain family resources and place especially huge demands on hospital beds, rehabilitation and social work support services (Law *et al.* 1991). The postmenopausal woman is characterised in terms of her potential liability and also her (un)willingness to protect others from her own needs for care. A degenerating postmenopausal woman is constructed as an object of public interest who can be harangued into submitting to numerous preventive medicine strategies. Striving for invulnerability is made a normative condition of appropriate older womanhood. Individualised treatment through the use of HRT is offered as a solution to the political problems of caring for others (for example, husbands and grand-children), the availability of adequate hospital care in the event of fracture and the modifications to homes, streets, public building and transport facilities which may help guard against accidents leading to fractures. Medical authors construct a desiring position of subjectivity for the postmenopausal woman in which she desires to be useful and not burden others, and therefore desires therapies and interventions which are capable of conferring greater personal value. They assume that, at an individual level, health, fitness and independence are meaningful and attainable goals.

Women's health texts construct fitness as an object of desire for menopausal women and emphasise the importance of women's health for themselves. They make the political point that women can attain health and fitness through self-help which constitutes '*real* prevention' and a way of 'wrestling control *for* the consumer, *away* from the medical system and makers of highly profitable products' (Worcester and Whately 1992: 23). Feminist women's health writers have argued against preventing osteoporosis and cardiovascular disease with HRT on the grounds that they are 'lifestyle diseases'. Instead, they argue for a 'healthy lifestyles' approach to disease prevention, which includes adopting 'natural, safer, healthier and less expensive' alternative therapies and 'changing harmful practices' (like stopping smoking and decreasing alcohol, caffeine and total fat intake) and 'helping ourselves' through regular weight-bearing exercise and dietary changes[9] (National Women's Health Network 1989: 7).

However, a 'healthy lifestyle' approach to health and the designation of harmful practices (as a means of preventing disease and gaining control over one's life) implies that women who smoke, do not exercise or who eat fatty diets are not helping themselves and are potentially out of control. This approach obscures the point that healthy lifestyle practices are defined within cultural relations which shape the horizons on which different individuals act as part of their capacities to act

(Butler 1992). These include having money, time and access to facilities which make it possible and desirable to eat a particular diet and exercise. The regulative effects of health promotion through self-help, like medical characterisations of disease prevention, include the articulation of an obligation to pursue health, the stipulation of the terms and conditions under which health can be pursued and the exclusion of those for whom each condition represents a point of irrelevancy or failure.

Joanne Finkelstein has argued that individuals have tacitly agreed, as a condition of being normal, acceptable members of society, to being surveyed and measured by a calculating medical eye (Finkelstein 1990: 14). Increasingly, she argues, the value of a person will be measured by his or her capacities which may include the performance of certain physical and mental tasks and even the capacity to resist specific illnesses (Finkelstein 1990: 15). An emphasis on sex-linked mortality and morbidity rates in discourses constructing HRT suggests concern about lost usefulness. Indeed, in an era of economic rationalism, these emphases may simply be an extension of a major contemporary and all-pervasive 'discourse on productivity', which stresses, above all else, individuals' capacity to be productive. HRT, constructed as an active strategy against death and debility, may operate to constitute an emphasis on the value of older women judged according to their capacity to resist degenerative diseases, to appear fit and youthful, to function independently and to be available to care for others. By the same token, diseases like osteoporosis and cardiovascular disease are made to exhaust all possible significations of the postmenopausal woman thus diagnosed. It is conceivable that not using HRT may become a comment on an individual woman's sense of responsibility to self and community. The idea that HRT may prevent osteoporosis or cardiovascular disease may make for less tolerance of women disabled by these diseases if they have not taken HRT. They may be perceived as a financial burden on the community (Finkelstein 1990: 15). Further, the argument that hormonal therapy is more relevant to some women, especially 'thin white women' (Marsh and Whitehead 1992: 431), and its lack of availability to others (who may be neither offered nor able to afford treatment) guarantee that deployment of HRT will render white middle-class women responsible, and (through their exclusion) work-ing-class and black women careless and a burden on welfare systems. Women's health discourse which emphasises alternative means of pursuing health also places the onus on the individual to pursue health, even though some writers recognise that many older women may be constrained by the social circumstances (like poverty) in which they live (Coney 1991; Klein 1992).

In each discourse, through the excitement of desires for 'invulnerability' and 'health', individuals are recruited into practices directed at disease avoidance. Productivity and usefulness are rendered major reference points for individuals. Health is produced as a cultural defence against an encroaching 'other' and paramount cultural value (a resource or capacity) of relevance to each individual. The political significance of this conceptualisation of health is that it is formulated as a series of common endpoints for groups and individuals, obscuring their sheer impossibility for some.

In various ways, medical and feminist discourses converge in their use of a discourse on risk and emphases on surveillance and health promotion, albeit under the auspices and control of different agents. Medical and feminist constructions of the postmenopausal woman (sick or well) also rest on similar assumptions about the reliability of the category 'sex' as a prior and firm basis for their different claims to truth. Each presumes the prior arrangement of bodies as sexed in detailing their risks of succumbing to diseases like cardiovascular disease and breast cancer and in advocating that women exercise control over their bodies.

MEDICALISATION

Feminist writers on women's health have criticised the medicalisation of women's lives, whereby 'normal' and 'natural' physiological processes like menstruation, childbirth and menopause are defined as pathological and in need of treatment, on the grounds that medicalisation contributes to women's subjugation (Zita 1988; Martin 1989; Coney 1991; Klein 1992; Worcester and Whately 1992).[10] This line of argument produces a medicalised body and, conversely, an unmedicalised/natural body. It also promotes oppositions between clinical and everyday discourse, men and women. This strategy also constitutes women patients or potential patients as a homogeneous group, with common interests and relations to clinical encounters, symptom narratives, men and idealised, unmedicalised lives. It constructs a singular female body based on common experience of 'normal physiological processes'. It does not easily take account of how relations of power shape the different subject positions from which women may seek to negotiate or reject clinical verdicts and procedures, nor the subject positions excluded by a focus on the clinic and resistance to medical control.

In contrast, I suggest, owing to the medicalisation of life generally and the promulgation of medical statements about symptoms and diseases and their treatments, in the clinic and in the media, as news and entertainment, it is hard to isolate examples of medicalisation from its absences, and to distinguish a medicalised body from an unmedicalised body. Indeed, owing to the power of medical discourse to frame experience of bodily processes, the unmedicalised body is a sheer impossibility. Even individuals who, through lack of access to medical services, appear to escape medical scrutiny may be positioned by this absence. Indeed, they may be subject to censorship by others in the name of health promotion or disease prevention (for example, visibly pregnant women are sometimes cautioned by complete strangers against smoking). Medicalisation is an uneven enactment of bodily regulation, which does not discriminate only between women and men. The main problem with a feminist critique of medicalisation is that it fails to fully appreciate the huge extent to which bio-medical understandings permeate and dominate contemporary discourse on the body and provide the main framework through which bodies currently become culturally intelligible.

In many women's health texts, disease and sex are constructed as exclusive of each other and reproduction is seen as their major meeting point. In these texts, disease is produced as a site of negativity, reprisal and repression, where power flows only in one direction, exerted by medical experts over the generic woman patient. Medical observation and explanation are constituted as imposed on passive and unwilling bodies. Disease is a result of sexism which is secondary to and presupposes the coherence and fixity of an underlying sexed body. Further, a persistent challenge by women's health discourse to the diseasing of (normal) reproductive bodily processes, and insistence that these are not really diseases, implies that somewhere else there exist other 'real' diseases. (How) are these diseases related to sex? I suggest that it is possible to think of diseases not as being at home in a body that is already either male or female, but rather as being elements in the sexing and subjection of bodies.

SEX AND THE BODY IN DISCOURSES ON HRT

Within the critical domain of feminist discourse on women's health issues, the ontology of the natural body and the category 'sex' inscribed in medical discourse have not been questioned (Harding 1996). Rather than being radically different, medical and feminist discourses on HRT share several common assumptions. To begin with, both presuppose the reality of an underlying physiological body and its reproductive capacity, although they appear to interpret and invest it differently. Both medical and feminist constructions of a postmenopausal woman presuppose 'sex' as a fixed and permanent category, and a precondition for designating menopause and individuals requiring/not requiring treatment. In different ways, each discourse produces and depends upon the separation of a coherent and stable pre-existing female body from a more flexible and tentative femininity. Femininity is made available to modification through either bio-medical interventions or re-socialisation/emancipation. The female body, despite its being the malleable object of various transforming disciplinary practices (surgical, medical, cosmetic, dietary), and the site of their acceptance or rejection, is produced as the singular and intransigent site of both the biological determination and cultural construction of femininity and women, whereby it is assigned normal attributes and gains a certain visibility. Both medical and feminist discourses on HRT appear to position the female body as a constant substratum underpinning different (medicalised/unmedicalised) constructions of femininity and women (Harding 1993).

The female body is rendered a universal fact by virtue of being seen to be outside of, and prior to, history and culture. A universalised and naturalised version of the sexed body has been produced and perpetuated through medical discourse. This version of the body has also been maintained by feminists who demonstrate that gender is culturally constructed but do not also interrogate the ways in which the body is invested in culture and, in particular, the construction of anatomical differences upon which gender relations are built. This is in part the legacy of an historical distinction between sex and gender, in which it is argued that gender is not the result of a male or female body but is culturally constructed and therefore amenable to reconstruction within culture (Butler 1990a). Within the logic of the sex/gender distinction, sex poses as 'the real', material, corporeal base upon which 'gender operates as an act of cultural *inscription*' (Butler 1990a: 146; emphasis in original).

Feminist discourse on HRT and other women's health issues is problematic, I suggest, because it typically embraces the proposition that both unity and difference among women can be expressed in terms of their *experience* of their bodies. The female body is thereby produced as a stable entity denoting an 'integral otherness' which underpins women as a singular social positioning (Riley 1988). As others have pointed out, this production is normative and also politically limiting in that it has 'serious exclusionary implications' (Butler 1990b: 325).

FURTHER THOUGHTS

I am concerned that feminist women's health strategies on HRT lack sufficient critical edge to adequately challenge and transform the regulatory effects of medical discourse. Feminist women's health discourse is stymied by persistent assumptions about the stability of a female body and its capacity to designate an integral otherness uniting 'women' (Riley 1988: 105), and the continuing use of medical idiom and commitment to medically led research (National Women's Health Network 1989; Worcester and Whately 1992). Most texts fail to articulate clearly what they mean by 'healthy' and fail to recognise the regulatory effects of their attempts to normalise and naturalise menopause and extend and individualise consumer choices in health care. Women's health discourse needs to disengage from dominating discourses and to examine the local practices of power operating through medically nominated categories, like risk factors and disease labels, if it is to further transform relations of power.

Through their deployment of the construct 'risk', which fuels desire for health and disease prevention, medical and women's health discourses encourage women to make themselves objects of self-surveillance. The ageing woman's desire is circumscribed by a responsibility to resist her own decrepitude. This responsibility separates the vigilant from the non-vigilant, healthy and sick.

HRT can be viewed as a technology of power directed at bodies which establishes, at the level of the body, unequal distributions of power and thereby contributes to the manufacture of sexed subjects and the definition of conditions of being a sex. Sex can be seen as an effect of the investments in the body made possible by discourses, in this case on HRT, producing its natural and normal precondition and subsequent secondary characterisations.

NOTES

1 HRT has been considered controversial since the 1960s, when Robert Wilson vigorously promoted it for all women 'from menopause to the grave' and published his book *Feminine Forever* (1966), outlining the 'de-feminising' effects of oestrogen deficiency.

2 Some have cautioned against the potential dangers to women of a new technology of 'unproven' safety and benefit, in the light of the tragic consequences of previous medical interventions like the use of DES (an early version of oral oestrogen; see Lewis 1993) and 'Thalidomide' in pregnancy (Klein 1992: 28; Worcester and Whately 1992: 23).

3 Thus, 'there is no power relation without the correlative constitution of a field of knowledge, nor any knowledge, that does not presuppose and constitute at the same time power relations' (Foucault 1979: 27).

4 This conceptualisation does not involve denying a prediscursive existence for the subject or for the objects of discourse. Rather, whether or not object and subjects exist outside of discourse, they are constituted as such within discourse (Laclau and Mouffe 1985: 108). Within this framework, even their prediscursive existence is produced in discourse.

5 By 'medical discourse', I mean what is said by those speaking as medical experts, and which locates them as such, in a clinical setting, a lecture hall or on the printed page. I use the term 'women's health discourse' to refer to discursive strategies which are in some way associated, however loosely, with each other through the term 'feminist'. Discontinuities in the constitution and deployment of feminist assumptions and ideas are glaringly apparent. I deliberately concentrate on themes in common in order to characterise an emerging discursive field. Women's health strategies have in common the aims of diminishing medical control over women's bodies and transferring (variable degrees of) control to women and have spawned a significant women's health 'movement' (Haug 1987: 247). They seek to offer women a basis from which to evaluate and take up, or seek alternatives to, medical treatments. Women's health discourses mainly focus on objects already formulated as objects of medical interest, like menopause, pre-menstrual syndrome, management of childbirth and fertility control. However, in seeking to articulate statements from positions which challenge medical discourse, women's health discourses differ from other practices formulating 'women's health issues', like community-based menopause clinics, which construct women's health as a sub-specialism within the organisation of established medical services. There are examples of this in UK menopause clinics, run by general practitioners, and in clinics run by community nurses in Victoria, Australia. Women's health discourses may be articulated from outside of state or privately run health care services.

6 An editorial in *The Lancet* stated that despite well-established benefits, including symptom relief and disease prevention, only 9 per cent of postmenopausal women in London and 3 per cent in Glasgow receive HRT for more than 3 years. Even where HRT was prescribed there was little long-term use, beyond a few months (*The Lancet* 1991: 917).

7 Thus, for each round of clinically produced adverse effects, a new round of drugs is prescribed and pharmaceutical solutions found (Illich 1977: 82). Authors foreclose the possibility that the failure of one medication might compromise trust in another.

8 Depending on the health care system (which varies between countries) women may have to pay for assessment and treatment for menopausal symptoms. Black women are claimed to be less at risk of osteoporosis than other women (Marsh and Whitehead 1992: 432). The designation 'white' to describe the body most at risk constitutes the subject whom clinicians are preparing to protect.

9 Weight-bearing exercise includes walking, bicycle riding, aerobics, jogging and workouts. Dietary changes include increasing intake of calcium, vitamin D and vegetables and fruit.

10 Jacqueline Zita conceptualises 'medicalisation' (in her analysis of the emergence of pre-menstrual syndrome [PMS]) as a process whereby 'subjectively expressed meanings voiced by women' are codified into 'quantifiable symptoms and signs' sharing a common pattern of pre-menstrual cyclicity (Zita 1988: 85–6). The medicalised female body, constituted as an object of interest for the medical gaze, is removed from the social and ideological contexts in which it is lived and interpreted. It is problematised as 'an aggregate of clinically detectable organic or psychogenic events' for which causes are located within its boundaries (Zita 1988: 90). Thus, clinical discourse provides objective and scientific legitimation for sexist interpretations of women's bodies and actions in everyday discourse, where negative evaluations and 'complaints' requiring medical redefinition are formulated (Zita 1988: 85–6).

REFERENCES

Butler, J. (1990a) *Gender Trouble. Feminism and the Subversion of Identity*, New York and London: Routledge.
Butler, J. (1990b) 'Gender trouble, feminist theory, and psychoanalytic discourse', in L. Nicholson (ed.) *Feminism/Postmodernism*, New York and London: Routledge.
Butler, J. (1992) 'Contingent foundations: feminism and the question of "postmodernism"', in J. Butler and J. Scott (eds) *Feminists Theorize the Political*, New York and London: Routledge.
Coney, S. (1991) *The Menopause Industry: A Guide to Medicine's 'Discovery' of the Mid-life Woman*, Auckland: Penguin Books.
Finkelstein, J. (1990) 'Bio-medicine and technocratic power', *Hastings Center Report*, 20, 4: 13–16.
Foucault, M. (1979) *Discipline and Punish: The Birth of the Prison*, New York: Vintage Books.
Foucault, M. (1981) *The History of Sexuality, Volume I: An Introduction*, Harmondsworth, Middlesex: Penguin Books.
Foucault, M. (1986) *The Archaeology of Knowledge*, London: Tavistock.
Goldman, L. and Tosteson, A. (1991) 'Uncertainty about postmenopausal estrogen', editorial, *The New England Journal of Medicine*, 235, 11: 800–2.
Gorman, T. and Whitehead, M. (1989) *The Amarant Book of Hormone Replacement Therapy*, London: Pan Books.
Greer, G. (1991) *The Change: Women, Ageing and the Menopause*, London: Hamish Hamilton.
Harding, J. (1993) 'Regulating sex: constructions of the postmenopausal woman in discourses on hormone replacement therapy', unpublished PhD thesis, University of Technology, Sydney.
Harding, J. (1996) 'Sex and control: the hormonal body', *Body and Society*, 2 (1): 99–111.
Haug, F. (ed.) (1987) *Female Sexualization: A Collective Work of Memory*, London: Verso.
Illich, I. (1977) *Limits to Medicine. Medical Nemesis: The Exploration of Health*, Harmondsworth, Middlesex: Pelican Books.

Klein, R. (1992) 'The unethics of hormone replacement therapy', *Bioethics News*, 11, 3: 24–37.

Laclau, E. and Mouffe, C. (1985) *Hegemony and Socialist Strategy: Towards a Radical Democratic Politics*, London: Verso.

The Lancet (1991) 'More than hot flushes', editorial, *The Lancet*, 338: 917–18.

Law, M., Wald, N. and Meade, T. (1991) 'Strategies for prevention of osteoporosis and hip fracture', *British Medical Journal*, 303: 453–9.

Lewis, J. (1993) 'Feminism, the menopause and hormone replacement therapy', *Feminist Review*, 43: 38–56.

Long Hall, D. (1973) 'Biology, sex hormones and sexism in the 1920s', *Philosophical Forum*, 5, 1–2: 81–96.

Lupton, D. (1995) *The Imperative of Health: Public Health and the Regulated Body*, London: Sage Publications.

MacLennan, A. (1991) 'Hormone replacement therapy and the menopause', *Medical Journal of Australia*, 155: 43–4.

MacLennan, A. (1992) 'Menopause and preventive medicine', editorial, *Australian Family Physician*, 21, 3: 205.

Marsh, M. and Whitehead, M. (1992) 'Management of the menopause', *British Medical Bulletin*, 48, 2: 426–57.

Martin, E. (1989) *The Woman in the Body: A Cultural Analysis of Reproduction*, Milton Keynes: Open University Press.

Moon, T. (1991) 'Estrogens and disease prevention', editorial, *Archives of Internal Medicine*, 151: 17–18.

National Women's Health Network (1989) *Taking Hormones and Women's Health: Choices, Risks and Benefits*, Washington: National Women's Health Network.

Oudshoorn, N. (1994) *Beyond the Natural Body. An Archaeology of Sex Hormones*, London and New York: Routledge.

Riley, D. (1988) *'Am I that Name?' Feminism and the Category of 'Women' in History*, London: Macmillan Press.

Stampfer, M., Colditz, G., Willett, W. *et al.* (1991) 'Postmenopausal estrogen therapy and cardiovascular disease. Ten-year follow-up from the Nurses' Health Study', *New England Journal of Medicine*, 325, 11: 756–62.

Treichler, P. (1987) 'AIDS, homophobia and bio-medical discourse: an epidemic of signification', *Cultural Studies*, 1, 3, pp. 263–305.

Vines, G. (1993) *Raging Hormones: Do They Rule Our Lives?*, London: Virago.

Wilson, R. (1966) *Feminine Forever*, New York: M. Evans.

Worcester, N. and Whately, M. (1992) 'The selling of HRT: playing on the fear factor', *Feminist Review*, 41: 1–26.

Wren, B. (1992) 'HRT and the cardiovascular system', *Australian Family Physician*, 21, 3: 226–9.

Zita, J. (1988) 'The pre-menstrual syndrome: "dis-easing" the female cycle', *Hypatia*, 3, 1: 157–68.

Chapter 8

Foucault, embodiment and gendered subjectivities
The case of voluntary self-starvation

Liz Eckermann

> From the idea that the self is not given to us, I think that there is only
> one practical consequence, we have to create ourselves as a work of art.
>
> (Foucault 1983: 237)

THE SELF AS WORK OF ART

The person who voluntarily starves uses her body to recreate herself.
She recreates herself 'as a work of art' whose bodily form is so
confronting that it cannot be, and is not, ignored. The message
conveyed by the emaciated self-starver is: 'Read my body!'

Place (1989: 268), an 'ex-sufferer of anorexia nervosa', describes
her experience thus:

> she twitched
> and twitched
> longed for some
> understanding
> for the words.

But the words did not come. She recalls:

> the battle to find words to express the world as it is – full of
> paradoxes and not the narrow, simple place some parents describe it
> to be.
>
> (Place 1989: 268)

The classical and modern traditions of sociology have little to
contribute in understanding such messages since they are largely
disembodied traditions which rely on evidence from the rational
reflexive mind expressed through the spoken and written word. In the

mainstream classical and modern traditions there are no spatial and temporal concepts to allow analysis of such phenomena, much less a sociology of the body. When interviewees say 'There are no words to describe how I feel' and they answer questions with poems or bodily gestures – where is mainstream sociology's explanatory power?

I suggest that phenomenology, post-structuralism and postmodernism provide the theoretical means to deconstruct embodied communication. In this chapter I will concentrate on the contributions that a Foucauldian analysis offers to understanding the contradictory discourses of self-starvation. I argue that Foucault's analysis of the development of disciplinary society helps to explain the conditions for the rise of an epidemic of self-starvation in the late twentieth century and that his later work on power as constitutive and the self as agent aids an understanding of self-starvation as resistance.

The message conveyed by the emaciated body is contradictory. It acts as a parody of disciplinary society to which the self-starver is the super-compliant servant or the 'secular saint' (if we all ate less fat, less sugar and less salt, we too could be 'thin'). At the same time self-starvation defies both the dictates of science (if you don't eat you die, yet the self-starver is still alive) and the authority of parents, teachers and the medical profession in a search for independent selfhood.

BEYOND THE CLASSICAL AND MODERN

Foucault challenges all of the underpinnings of what passes for 'modern', most especially the unitary standpoint in relation to theory and the concept of the 'self' and the implications of this unitary theoretical framework in relation to power and possibilities for effective social change. McNay (1992: 1) summarises the questions that many sociologists raise about the political implications of adopting a Foucauldian theoretical framework to understand social phenomena, thus:

> Firstly, where does the post-structuralist deconstruction of unified subjectivity into fragmented subject positions lead in terms of an understanding of individuals as active agents capable of intervening in and transforming their social environment? Secondly, what are the implications of the postmodern suspension of all forms of value judgement, of concepts such as truth, freedom and rationality, for emancipatory political projects?

In answer to the first question, my research interviewing young women who self-starve suggests that political agendas are not compromised by using Foucault to understand voluntary starvation. If anything, post-structuralism sheds light on the extent to which a search for selfhood (and independence) exists alongside a pursuit of secular 'sainthood' ('goodness' in secular terms) in many self-starvers' constructions of themselves. The second question raised by Foucault's critics, when applied to self-starvation, addresses the issue: 'Is self-starvation a problem?' and 'if so, whose problem?' Are there conditions under which it is rational to starve oneself? What if self-starvation is seen as a solution rather than a problem by the self-starver? I will deal with the first question raised by the critics of post-structuralism and then explore the implications of suspended notions of truth and rationality.

FRAGMENTED SUBJECT POSITIONS

Much modern sociological theory rests on an acceptance of the concept of the universality of a search for integration in individuals' beliefs, attitudes, values and actions. This is seen for instance in the work of Festinger (1957) in his theory of 'cognitive dissonance'. The theory of dissonance is based on the assumption that the individual 'strives towards consistency within himself [sic] . . . the existence of dissonance, being psychologically uncomfortable, will motivate the person to try to reduce the dissonance and to achieve consonance' (Festinger 1957: 1–3). In sociological theory this concept is generalised to the social system as evidenced in the homeostatic theme of Parsons's arguments in *The Social System* (1951). The pursuit of harmony also underlies Giddens's (1991) claim that the project of the self involves the production of a 'coherent 'and 'unitary' self. In fact, the notion of people being motivated by a search for personal consistency and integrity has inhered in much social theory since the Enlightenment.

Foucault denies unitary theoretical constructs and the search for 'internal consistency' and argues for the need to adopt a de-centred approach to both individual identity and social formations. Thus any given individual, and any particular society, can contain multiple, shifting and often self-contradictory identities. Added to this is the concept that there is no way of judging the value of one of those identities over the others. There are, as Foucault argues, 'many ways of being'. It is this recognition of the many ways of being that renders Foucault more useful than Giddens (1991, 1992) in understanding voluntary self-starvation, since literature on self-starvation over the last decade (Bordo 1988; Probyn 1988; Robertson 1992; Eckermann 1994) has identified contradictory, shifting and multiple identities amongst those who starve themselves.

TWO FOUCAULTS? THE DOCILE VERSUS THE ACTIVE SELF

Foucault's theorising about power goes through several major transformations over the course of his writing career. His earlier works on institutions, such as his analysis of asylums (1965) and the clinic (1973), the hospital (1973), the prison (1979) and public health (1980), emphasise external constraints on the power of individuals via the disciplines. Both Patton (1989) and McNay (1992) document the transformation which occurred in Foucault's conception of power in the early 1980s. In his later work, from the first volume of *History of Sexuality* (1981) onward, Foucault offers a framework to theorise the self which allows for the exercise of individual agency. It is this latter emphasis in Foucault's work which has been ignored by many of his critics (Patton 1989; McNay 1992).

Foucault's early works on the production of docile subjects and his later writing on the active self, as elaborated in volumes two and three of *The History of Sexuality* (*The Use of Pleasure* and *The Care of the Self*), prove singularly fertile in providing conceptual tools for understanding the body from a sociological perspective and specifically for gaining insights into the historical forces behind the modern 'epidemic' of self-starvation. His ideas have also formed the focus of new therapeutic techniques for dealing with such 'disorders', and these techniques specifically apply Foucault's 'general spectrum of power' (White and Epston 1989).

White and Epston note the use of analyses of power in therapy literature as traditionally representing power 'in individual terms such as a biological phenomenon that affects the individual psyche' or as 'individual pathology that is the inevitable outcome of early traumatic experience' (White and Epston 1989: 25). They identify attempts to apply Marxist class analysis in terms of power in the relations of production and 'a number of feminist analyses of the operation of power . . . as a gender-specific repressive phenomenon' which they see as having 'sensitized many therapists to the gender-related experience of abuse, exploitation and oppression'. However they argue that 'it is important to consider the more general spectrum of power as well, not just its repressive aspects, but also its constitutive aspects'; thus the work of Michel Foucault is important (White and Epston 1989: 25).

Foucault's work on the disciplined society provides an analysis of the connectedness of the body, self and society, thus combining the macro and micro traditions of sociological analysis (Silverman 1985). Although his earlier work minimises the role of agency and the 'self', he refers to the politico-anatomy of the body and the bio-politics of the society as being inseparable parts of the general exercise of power. One of Turner's (1984, 1987, 1992) unique contributions to a sociology of the body in extending Foucault's analysis is to draw parallels between regimes of given societies and the regimes people apply to their own bodies. An administered society develops in response to the fact that all societies are confronted by four tasks, namely: the reproduction of population in time, the regulation of bodies in space, restraint of the interior body through disciplines and representation of the exterior body in social space (Turner 1984: 91). Self-starvation, and the ascetic practices that accompany it, reflect the overlap between these levels of administration. Self-starvation may represent a personal solution to a broader social problem of lack of order and control. This process is also normalised in the self-starvation that accompanies World Vision's 40-Hour Famine, whereby ascetic practices of starvation at an individual level are used to appease social guilt about structural inequality globally.

Foucault uses language as a key variable in explaining how social power is exercised, and how social relations of class, gender and race can be transformed. Foucault's place in this tradition is unique in his insistence on the importance of historical processes and specific 'moments' as heuristic devices in gaining insight into present social processes. In arguing that language circumscribes social reality, Foucault suggests that one should direct one's attention to the specific details of the discursive field which constitute concepts such as body, illness and madness at a particular historical moment, in the service of gaining understanding of how particular power/knowledge processes are at work (Place 1989; Ussher 1991).

MEDICALISATION AND OBJECTIFICATION OF BODIES

Foucault's analyses (1979, 1981) of the medicalisation and objectivisation of the persons of 'marginal groups' in the seventeenth century and the subsequent hysterisation of women's bodies in the eighteenth century (1981) are of particular relevance to understanding self-starvation and binge-purging. The disciplining of the body and the self-denying regime evident in the self-starving individual can be related to the historical process of objectivisation of bodies.

With the development of the Hôpital Générale in Paris in 1656, the poor, the prostitutes, the vagabonds and the 'insane' were rounded up, institutionalised and subjected to a series of experiments, controls and surveillance. The development of the idea and practices of treating individuals as objects can be observed in this situation. 'Marginal' groups were excluded from the population at large, from the mainstream of culture, a process which had started with the exclusion of lepers. Thus these groups were given an identity by the majority group as 'outcasts' and the use of the word 'leper' as a metaphor for 'outcasts' emerged. Such 'outcasts' were seen as not meeting the criterion of being persons.

The second stage of the objectivisation process was that bodies were treated as objects. Foucault argued that 'the study of human beings took a decisive turn' at the end of the eighteenth century. 'Human beings came to be interpreted as knowing subjects and at the same time as objects of their own knowledge' (Foucault 1981). With the development of epidemiology, statistical techniques for aggregating social data, clinical medicine and the application of science to the social sphere, bodies could be transformed into objects. Women were especially vulnerable to this process because the traditional areas of female medical knowledge and therapeutic techniques did not fit the requirements and specifications of scientific medicine. Women were ascribed a specific identity by men and relegated to the spheres of nature, emotion, desire and the household. Women's knowledge in the area of birthing and healing was undermined by the application of clinical medicine with its instrumental-rational base. The objectivisa-tion of the body in self-starvation is reflected in the development of the thin body as a project to be worked upon. Similarly, the binge-purging body becomes an object to be 'filled up' and 'emptied'. Thus it could be argued that the stage was set long ago for the development of contemporary self-starvation and binge-purging (White 1988).

'Rational' developments in other fields such as architecture came with the emergence of modern medicine. Foucault (1979) notes the application within institutionalised settings (especially the prison and the hospital) of an architectural design which reflected the develop-ments in science of techniques of control and surveillance – this covered control and surveillance of whole populations (census data, epidemiology, registers of demographic data) and surveillance of bodies (with developments in clinical medicine and anatomy). The design emanated from Jeremy Bentham's notion of the Panopticon which involved maximum supervision with minimum effort (Foucault 1980;

Armstrong 1983). The Panopticon's 'potential' for surveillance nurtures self-discipline (causing individuals to 'gaze upon themselves') and self-discipline replaces torture as the 'paradigmatic' method of social control. Thus where persons themselves and their bodies are turned into 'objects', self-surveillance emerges as a practice of control. This practice is reflected in language ('Watch yourself'), architecture and power relations. When people are treated as objects they see themselves as objects and tend to torture their bodies and desires to fit instructions and specifications. They evaluate their own behaviour and tend to become either docile subjects or rebellious subjects. The self-starvers whom I interviewed as part a major study on self-starvation and binge purging (Eckermann 1994) displayed both of these extremes. Sandy talked of the:

> power I felt when asked by Dr K. to register on the body size metre how large I thought I was. As I moved the lever a ridiculous distance out I watched his reaction from the corner of my eye. His expression was 'Boy this kid is wacko!' and all the time I knew what I was doing manipulating him and it gave me enormous pleasure.

At the other extreme Tammy desperately wanted to please. She wanted to be 'super-good, not to cause anyone any fuss' and argued that over time she 'felt anything anyone thought [she] should feel and became everything [she perceived] her parents, her teachers and her friends thought she should become'. She believes her self-starving started when she could 'no longer read the messages of how [she] ought to be'. Both of these examples suggest that self-starvation represents defiance of prescriptions of 'normality' but in Tammy's case such a response followed years of absolute conformity as a docile subject.

Ironically a modification of the Panopticon architectural design is adopted in the large hospitals where self-starvers are treated. The concept of surveillance and the production of docile subjects are central to the treatment process in treatment regimes based on behaviour modification. The point of the exercise is to break the self-starver's will. In my study, the rooms chosen for those undergoing behaviour modification were within sight of the nurses' station, with glass panels internally and large windows to the outside to allow uninterrupted vision. All meals, showers and toileting were carefully supervised. Despite this level of surveillance, many of my interviewees, who had been institutionalised under such a regime, boasted of their ability to dispose of food or to exercise undetected. In one instance the 'patient' was able to deposit much of the food presented to her into the hollow steel tubular bed head, even while under the eagle eye of the nurse who supervised her eating. The hiding place was only detected weeks later when foul smells emanated from her room. Thus the tension between striving for 'sainthood' by keeping the body need-free and thus morally unsullied and the drive for selfhood in defying the dictates of authorities comes to a head in the therapeutic setting. Turner (1992: 221) succinctly encapsulates this dilemma in suggesting that:

> The anorexic avoids the shameful world of eating, while simultaneously achieving personal power and a sense of moral superiority through the emaciated body. Their attempt at disembodiment through negation becomes the symbol of their moral empowerment.

Over time the specification of 'normality' has become narrower and more stringent – it is easier to fall outside of the specifications where the penalties are harsh (institutionalisation). Self-maximisation, self-actualisation, self-discovery in psychology and in community services are emphasised. Thus to qualify as a 'normal' person one must torture oneself in relation to strict and constricting criteria (in both mind and body). Language is an important part of this process of self-evaluation and self-monitoring. Concepts like 'insight', 'guilt', 'hang-ups', 'obsessions' are used as people operate on themselves to test their existence against 'normality'.

The implications for women are enormous, given their continuing marginal social status. In the narrowing specifications of how women should be, women operate within the language of patriarchy and consumerism which forms the dominant discourse of twentieth-century society. The self-starving and binge-purging individuals who emerge in such a society understand themselves in terms of these dominant discourses. Clara, whom I interviewed, claimed: 'I wear tent dresses to hide a multitude of sins!' These actions were designed to disguise the fact that she is not a secular 'saint'. However, as the examples cited above indicate, self-starvation can be seen as either super-conformity to or super-defiance of such dominant discourses.

Asceticism represents an aspect of objectivisation of bodies and self-surveillance of bodies. At the same time consumerism promotes the commoditisation of the body. Thus, it could be argued that the dominant discourse surrounding these processes determines, or at least circumscribes, the very consciousness of those who develop problems with eating. However, Celermajer (1987) argues that these processes only determine in a negative way the form of rebellion chosen by young women.

The argument that women tend to conform is put forward by Spitzack (1987), who employs Foucault's concepts of confession and surveillance to analyse the 'discourse of weight loss'. She argues that:

> weight-reducing techniques weave the language of science, deviance and theology to find the perpetuation of a wholly transparent female subject. The weight-conscious woman is divided within herself (mind versus body) and must ironically become and remain body-conscious to alleviate body consciousness.
>
> (1987: 357)

Foucault's analysis of the extent to which bodies are 'inscribed in discursive practice' provides a framework to understand how the dogma of weight-reducing discourse (which is legitimated in public health campaigns) problematises the body, especially the female body, which is seen as in need of alteration both by the 'owner' of the body and by medical and public health institutions through the medical gaze (Spitzack 1987: 357). Spitzack's analysis suggests that the use of Foucault's framework of discursive power can turn a self-induced 'disease' category into a political issue. 'Surveillance of the self plays a central role in domination strategies' (Spitzack 1987: 362) which constitute weight-reducing discourse. The individual views her body as 'ultimately untrustworthy' and its desires as 'capable of taking her over'. As Foucault explains, the separation of mind and body:

> permit[s] individuals to effect, by their own means, a certain number of operations on their bodies, their own souls, their own thoughts, their own conduct, and this in a manner so as to transform themselves, modify themselves, and to attain a certain state of perfection, happiness, purity, supernatural power.
>
> (1981: 367)

Spitzack (1987: 357–8) concludes that will-power (mind over matter) 'in the discourse of weight reduction, is a central component in the perpetuation of an obese population' and points to the paradox that despite the fact that 'American consumers spend an estimated ten billion dollars annually on reducing formulas' the 'failure rate among dieters is 98%'.

The decision to diet entails dissatisfaction with bodily appearance, which is so widespread amongst women as to be viewed as endemic (*Cleo* 1988; Ben Tovim and Morton 1989). Similarly 'the struggle between body and consumption' appears 'endemic to contemporary culture' and the 'metaphors of discipline and theology intertwine to establish a context of [social] disease centred on the Body' (Spitzack 1987: 359). Foucault's contributions to an understanding of these phenomena are considerable since his theoretical understanding of the self allows for multiple constitution of the self.

THE HYSTERICAL BODY

One of the ways in which women's bodies were given meaning and their selves made 'nervous' from the turn of the eighteenth century onwards was by the process of hysterisation, which involved:

> a three-fold process whereby the feminine body was analysed – qualified and disqualified – as being thoroughly saturated with sexuality; whereby it was integrated into the sphere of medical practices, by reason of a pathology intrinsic to it; whereby, finally, it was placed in organic communication with the social body (whose regulated fecundity it was supposed to ensure), the family space (of which it had to be a substantial and functional element), and the life of children (which it produced and had to guarantee, by virtue of a biologico-moral responsibility lasting through the entire period of the children's education): the Mother, with her negative image of 'nervous woman' constituted the most visible form of hysterisation.
>
> (Foucault 1981: 104)

Turner (1984: 183) claims that the 'historical specificity of the eruption of anorexia in the late nineteenth century' suggests a correlation between Foucault's idea of the 'hysterisation of women's bodies . . . and the peculiar conjunction of social structures which produced a crisis in middle-class urban family life. This conjunction of circumstances was combined with a specific interest in family organisation by the medical profession.'

TRUTH CONSTRUCTION AROUND THE STARVING BODY

Foucault saw the development of psychoanalysis as a further repression of the self rather than as 'a liberating step beyond the human sciences'. To Foucault (1981: 67), psychoanalysis was the 'culmination of a normalising confessional technology' first used by the early Catholic Church and which ensured that 'sex' as well as the 'body' became medicalised, psychiatrised, psychologised and hygienised. One could enter the 'illness' world and 'disordered' world via a variety of 'new personages':

the nervous woman, the frigid wife, the indifferent mother – or
worse the mother beset by murderous obsessions . . . the hysterical
or neurasthenic girl, the precocious and already exhausted child . . .

(Foucault 1981: 110)

Surveillance of the family under the gaze of the new professionals of
psychiatry and psychology could turn up a variety of ways of 'disturbed
being'. Foucault (1981: 111) argues that the family from the mid-
nineteenth century was compliant in this process:

> the family broadcast the long complaint of its sexual sufferings to
> doctors, educators, psychiatrists, priests and pastors, to all the
> experts who would listen . . . [it] engaged in searching out the
> slightest forces of sexuality in its midst, wrenching from itself the
> most difficult confession, soliciting an audience with everyone who
> might know something about the matter and opening itself
> unreservedly to endless examination.

This situation culminated in the late twentieth century in the rise of
family therapy as the procedure for tapping the dark recesses of
neurosis and psychosis, and from Freud onwards the tendency was to
blame the development of 'disorders' on inadequate parenting when no
biological cause for the 'illness process' could be discerned. The body,
and its sexuality, were problems at the middle level of analysis – the
family. With the 'long campaign of inoculation and vaccination went a
new emphasis on the family as the most constant agent of
medicalisation' (Foucault 1980: 172–3) and in explanations of anorexia
nervosa, from the nineteenth century onwards, the family emerges as a
key culprit (Turner 1990).

However, hygiene on the middle level in the family (and on the
micro-level of the individual) was supplemented with a grander
programme as the development of 'homo hygienicus' involved 'a
regime of health for [whole] populations [that entailed a certain number
of authoritarian medical interventions and controls] . . . the city with its
spatial variables [came to appear] as a medicalisable object' (Foucault
1980: 175). Foucault suggests that a 'different project was also
involved, that of the indefinite extension of strength, vigour, health and
life' at a more macro-level in the service of the economy, especially the
dominance of the bourgeoisie.

The emphasis on the body should undoubtedly be linked to the
process of growth and establishment of bourgeois hegemony: not,

however, because of the market value assumed by labour capacity, but because of what the 'cultivation' of its own body could represent politically, economically and historically for the present and the future of the bourgeoisie.

(Foucault 1981: 125)

However, Foucault goes on to suggest that it was 'a physical matter as well'.

The works published in great numbers at the end of the eighteenth century, on body hygiene, the art of longevity, ways of having healthy children and of keeping them alive as long as possible, and methods for improving the human lineage, bear witness to the fact: they thus attest to the correlation of this concern with the body and sex to a type of 'racism'.

(1981: 125)

One could speculate about the reasons for the interest in hygiene and healthy living inherent in the late twentieth-century world's obsession with health promotion (the second wave of emphasis on 'homo hygienicus'). The self-starving and/or binge-purging individual may represent a victim of such campaigns, given the dominant discourse which emerges surrounding the concept of healthy eating, healthy living, exercise and ascetic attention to lifestyle (Turner 1984; Kalucy 1987; Colquhoun 1989). If 'anorexia' represents slavish observance to the specifications of medical and public health discourse (whether such discourse is in the service of narrow professional interests or cost–benefit analysis for the state), its entrance into the realm of the 'abnormal' in relation to psychiatric categories is somewhat ironic. The normalising 'truth' that is constructed in the operation of power in relation to nutrition and 'lifestyle' has unintended consequences, such as obsessive concerns about weight, shape and eating.

Medical and psychiatric discourses act as definers of truth around the self-starving body. The almost universal use of the American Psychiatric Association's *Diagnostic and Statistical Manual* (currently DSM-IV), as an administrative process, attests to this. Laing (1988: 62) argued that DSM-III (APA 1985) functioned only as 'a billings list for third party payments. You have got to have an entry in DSM-III for the insurance company to pay up.' To be diagnosed as suffering from 'anorexia nervosa' or from 'bulimia', a person needs to fulfil the criteria set out in DSM-IV (APA 1994). There is an arbitrary cut-off point which decides whether you 'are in or not'. Psychiatrists emerge as key figures in an administered society, because they are in a position to define madness and disorders and their discourse pervades the rest of society.

Psychiatry has the power to influence discourse by being 'entrusted' to set the diagnostic criteria for 'madness' for the whole of society. By its arbitrary classifications, psychiatry is involved not only in imposing norms on people but also in providing the discourse through which people think; there appears a significant use of understanding of psychiatric concepts in the community generally. It has an influence on the way people 'can be'. Place (1989: 97) describes her experiences of the discourses around self-starving thus:

> The medical profession, under the guise of uniforming language for the purpose of clarity, adopts a language of clinical description. . . . The clinical discourse. . . . But language is never innocent. [Psychiatrists and the medical profession] use a language which denies sub-texts [and which]
>
>> refuses to flirt
>> to admit
>> to the hidden
>
> And it would seem to me that any language that denies sub-texts must be diminished in its capacity to effectively treat illness. Especially anorexia nervosa, which I believe is first and foremost a language problem.

Place (1989: 137) suggests that language and text are the appropriate sites for understanding self-starvation:

> The person with anorexia nervosa has, for various reasons, often failed to pick up the sub-texts of language that her/his peers use to decode the double meanings and messages given to them by parents, teachers and media.
>
> (Place 1989: 137)

Laing argues that DSM-III is 'very useful for controlling the population because you can bring [the criteria] to bear on practically anyone if the occasion seems to demand it . . . a mandate to strip anyone of their civil liberties' (Laing 1988: 61). Classifying and objectifying criteria in psychiatric medicine provide insurance companies with defined 'illnesses' on which to base their business. This presents a case of the extended medical gaze which may have a benign intent but some detrimental 'administering' and 'normalising' effects.

IMPLICATIONS FOR TRUTH CONTESTATION

Foucault's analysis emphasises that no power/knowledge is entirely dominant or ascendant over other discursive fields. The potential for the exercise of agency from within different discursive fields is always there, and this has significant repercussions for the development of alternative subjectivities and for countering the 'truth' generation which emanates from psychiatry.

> Let us not therefore ask why certain people want to dominate what they seek, what is their overall strategy. Let us ask, instead, how things work at the level of on-going subjugation, at the level of those continuous and uninterrupted processes which subject our bodies, govern our gestures, dictate our behaviours, etc. In other words . . . we should try to discover how it is that subjects are gradually, progressively, really and materially constituted through a multiplicity of organisms, forces, energies, materials, desires, thoughts etc. . . . We should try to grasp subjection in its material instance as constitution of subjects.
>
> (Foucault 1980: 97)

Foucault suggests that the process of constituting subjectivity occurs not 'top-down' but in circulatory ways whereby local power/knowledge processes are constitutive also. The individual, in this case the self-starver, can exercise agency not only in starting to eat again, but also by rewriting her problem of self-starvation (as defined by psychiatry and other institutions), as a solution to broader problems in her life.

Many critics of Foucault's arguments about power and language claim that while theoretically Foucault provides insight, the implications for political practice are sterile. If language constitutes all knowledge, how is deviance developed and sustained (Connell 1987; Turner 1987)? Similarly, given the nature of power and surveillance, how can one explain opposition, criticism and resistance to prevailing or dominant discourses? Foucault's epistemology makes it difficult to provide grounds for alternatives and a hiatus is evident between his theoretical accounts of society and their political implications. Furthermore, he is seen as ignoring subjective experience (Turner 1984, 1987).

Turner argues that Foucault, alone, provides us with a comprehensive framework for examining 'bodies in plural, that . . . is populations' (Turner 1992: 58). Against the charge of critics like Rorty (1986) and Taylor (1986) that Foucault's project is 'apolitical', it would seem that conceiving of bodies *en masse* is an inherently political exercise.

FOUCAULT AND POLITICAL PRACTICE

Weedon (1987) and McNay (1992) argue that Foucault's analysis is invaluable in developing a feminist political practice. Weedon suggests that what Foucault's work contributes to feminism is 'a contextualization of experience and an analysis of its constitution and ideological power':

> Although the subject in post-structuralism is socially constructed in discursive practices, she none the less exists as a thinking, feeling, subject and social agent capable of resistance and innovations produced out of the clash between contradictory subject positions and practices. She is also a subject able to reflect upon the discursive relations which constitute her and the society in which she lives and able to choose from the options available.
>
> (Weedon 1987: 125)

White and Epston's 'orientation in therapy . . . is considerably informed by Foucault's thought' (1989: 32). They suggest that Foucault's ideas provide them with tools with which to critique their 'own practices that are formed in the domain of power and knowledge':

> We would work to identify the context of ideas in which our practices are situated and would explore the history of those ideas. This would enable us to more readily identify the effects, dangers and limitations of these ideas and of our own practices . . . we would work to identify and critique those aspects of our work that might relate to the techniques of social control.
>
> (White and Epston 1989: 32–3)

These therapists see Foucault's concepts as being directly used in the service of clients.

> If we accept Foucault's proposal that the techniques of power that 'incite' persons to constitute their lives through 'truth' are developed and perfected at the local level and are taken up at the broader levels, then in joining with persons to challenge these practices, we would also accept that we are inevitably engaged in a political activity. This is not a political activity that involves the proposal of an alternative ideology, but one that challenges the techniques that subjugate persons to a dominant ideology.
>
> (White and Epston 1989: 33)

The specific techniques used to achieve this include 'externalisation' of the problem (that is, separating from the unitary knowledges), challenging techniques of power, such that 'docile bodies become enlivened spirits', resurrecting the subjugated knowledges, the generation of alternative stories and rewriting personal narratives (White and Epston 1989: 17–39). The above techniques White and Epston see as having particular relevance to treatment for self-starvation and binge-purging, which they believe 'reflect the pinnacle of achievement of [self-subjugating] power'. They suggest that there are many ways to 'know', that the dominant ways are historically specific and challengeable. They suggest that self-erasing stories can be rewritten as self-embracing stories.

Silverman (1985) is another writer who defends Foucault's project as a basis for practice. Silverman counters all three of the major critical charges against Foucault's work: Foucault's tendency to 'displace man', his relativism and his pessimism. Silverman argues that these criticisms represent a selective reading of Foucault's work. He suggests that Foucault offers a significant solution to the ongoing methodological problem of 'integrating macro and micro levels of analysis' (Silverman 1985: 91). Foucault provides both content and method for generating research and suggestions for therapeutic intervention.

In proposing 'existential ontological therapy' Foucault argues for the enabling role of language, alongside its restricting role in relation to its inadequacy in reflecting thought processes and feelings. He suggests that we can learn other ways of thinking and perceiving. However, they must occur on a broad basis, otherwise therapy can produce 'only isolated and temporary "areas" in which an individual's narrowing of reality may open up, while the contradictions and normalizing closure of our everyday social practices continue to produce individual problems and a general malaise' (Dreyfus 1987: 330). For Foucault, the effective agenda is to counteract the situation where:

> the individual, through a series of accidental historical interpreta-
> tions focussed on a series of paradigms, comes to have a one-
> dimensional, normalising understanding of reality in which every
> anomaly must finally be made to yield its truth and confirm (the
> individual's) systematic interpretation.
>
> (Dreyfus 1987: 330)

The implication is that all individuals are 'pathological' since they live in one dimension. The problems of the lack of language and lack of other dimensions of subjectivity to give expression to existence are taken up by the new feminist postmodernists and have particular relevance to self-starvers and binge-purgers. Foucault's analysis offers concrete treatment implications. Witness White and Epston's (1989) and Robertson's (1992) applications of Foucault to self-therapy.

CONCLUSION

Foucault also offers solutions to the other problems associated with traditional sociological understandings of self-starvation. His theories move beyond the media and the family, as institutions responsible for causing self-starvation, to look at discursive and non-discursive practices in all institutions of modern Western societies which regulate and control individuals. However, Foucault acknowledges, especially in his later work on the self (1986), the role of individual agency in determining outcomes. I agree with McNay's assessment that although Foucault's earlier work reduced social agents to docile and passive subjects, unable to act in an autonomous fashion, in the last two volumes of *The History of Sexuality* he does provide an 'elaboration of a notion of self' (McNay 1992: 3). Foucault also offers a theory of the body in social relations as the site of both negative and constitutive power and provides the most comprehensive account of the role of language in constructing illness and the body, both of which he conceives of as cultural rather than natural entities.

The self-starver is recreating a sense of self, but a self which is not based on a stylised notion of beauty. It is a self which is distant enough from our current culturally constructed notions of aesthetic beauty, 'outside the dictates of style', to not be merely a reflection of fashion. It appeals almost to the timeless image of the thirteenth-century Catholic saint or the Eastern ascetic rather than the twentieth-century fashion model. The self-starver challenges our sense of rationality and our twentieth-century Western sensibilities. Foucault's notions of the relativity of truth and the possibilities of multiple constitution of the self allow us to engage with these apparent anomalies rather than dismiss them as signs of irrational deviance.

REFERENCES

APA (American Psychiatric Association) (1985) *Diagnostic and Statistical Manual of Mental Disorders*, 3rd edn (DSM-III), Washington DC: APA.

APA (American Psychiatric Association) (1994) *Diagnostic and Statistical Manual of Mental Disorders*, 4th edn (DSM-IV), Washington DC: APA.

Armstrong, D. (1983), *Political Anatomy of the Body*, Cambridge: Cambridge University Press.

Ben Tovim, D. and Morton, J. (1989) *The Anorexia Nervosa and Bulimia Study Project*, Report to South Australian Health Commission.

Bordo, S. (1988) 'Anorexia nervosa – psychopathology as the crystallization of culture', in I. Diamond and L. Quinby (eds) *Feminism and Foucault; Reflections on Resistance*, Boston: Northeastern University Press.

Celermajer, D. (1987) 'Submission and rebellion: anorexia and a feminism of the body', *Australian Feminist Studies*, 5.

Cleo Magazine (1988) 'Fat is beautiful: but could advertising agencies make us believe it?', *Cleo*, August: 87–120.

Colquhoun, D. (1989) 'Healthism, the sociology of school knowledge and the curriculum', *TASA Conference*, Melbourne, December.

Connell, R.W. (1987) 'Scheherezade's children: critical reflections on Michel Foucault's *History of Sexuality*, Vol. 1', *Arena*, 78: 139–45.

Dreyfus, H.L. (1987) 'Foucault's critique of psychiatric medicine', *The Journal of Medicine and Philosophy*, 12, 4: 311–33.

Eckermann, E. (1994) 'Self-starvation and binge-purging: embodied selfhood/sainthood', *Australian Cultural History* (Special Issue on Bodies), 13: 82–99.

Festinger, L. (1957) *A Theory of Cognitive Dissonance*, London: Tavistock.

Foucault, M. (1965) *Madness and Civilization: A History of Insanity in the Age of Reason*, London: Tavistock.

Foucault, M. (1973) *The Birth of the Clinic: An Archaeology of Medical Perception*, New York: Pantheon Books.

Foucault, M. (1979), *Discipline and Punish: The Birth of the Prison*, Harmondsworth: Penguin.

Foucault, M. (1980) *Power/Knowledge*, edited by C. Gordon, London: Harvester.

Foucault, M. (1981) *The History of Sexuality: An Introduction*, London: Penguin.

Foucault, M. (1983) *M. Foucault: Beyond Structuralism and Hermeneutics*, 2nd edn, edited by H. Dreyfus and P. Rabinow, Chicago: University of Chicago Press.

Foucault, M. (1986) *The Foucault Reader*, edited by P. Rabinow, Harmondsworth: Penguin.

Foucault, M. (1987) *The History of Sexuality, Vol. 2: The Use of Pleasure*, London: Penguin.

Foucault, M. (1988), *The History of Sexuality, Vol. 3: The Care of the Self*, London: Penguin.

Giddens, A. (1991) *Modernity and Self-Identity: Self and Society in the Late Modern Age*, Stanford: Stanford University Press.

Giddens, A. (1992) *Transformation of Intimacy*, Cambridge: Polity Press.

Kalucy, R.S. (1987) 'The "new" nutrition', *The Medical Journal of Australia*, 147: 529–30.

Laing, R.D. (1988) 'Interview with R.D. Laing', Anthony Liversidge, *OMNI Magazine*, 10, 7: 56–63.

McNay, L. (1992) *Foucault and Feminism*, Cambridge: Polity Press

Parsons, T. (1951) *The Social System*, Glencoe, IL: Glencoe Free Press.

Patton, P. (1989) 'Taylor and Foucault on power and freedom', *Political Studies*, 37: 260–76.

Place, F. (1989) *Cardboard*, Sydney: Local Consumption Pubs.

Probyn, E. (1988) 'The anorexic body', in A. Kroker and M. Kroker (eds) *Body Invaders: Sexuality and the Postmodern Condition*, London: Macmillan.

Robertson, M. (1992) *Starving in the Silences: An Exploration of Anorexia Nervosa*, Sydney: Allen and Unwin.

Rorty, R. (1986) 'Foucault and epistemology', in D.C. Hoy (ed.) *Foucault: A Critical Reader*, Oxford: Basil Blackwell.

Silverman, D. (1985) *Qualitative Methodology and Sociology*, Aldershot: Gower.

Spitzack, C. (1987) 'Confessions and signification: the systematic inscription of body consciousness', *The Journal of Medicine and Philosophy*, 12, 4: 357–69.

Taylor, C. (1986) 'Foucault on freedom and truth', in D.C. Hoy (ed.) *Foucault: A Critical Reader*, Oxford: Basil Blackwell.

Turner, B.S. (1984) *The Body and Society*, Oxford: Basil Blackwell

Turner, B.S. (1987) *Medical Power and Social Knowledge*, London: Sage.

Turner, B.S. (1990) 'The talking disease: Hilda Bruch and anorexia nervosa', *Australian & New Zealand Journal of Sociology*, 26, 2: 157–69.

Turner, B.S. (1992) *Regulating Bodies: Essays in Medical Sociology*, London: Routledge.

Ussher, J. (1991) *Women's Madness: Misogyny or Mental Illness*, New York: Harvester Wheatsheaf.

Weedon, C. (1987) *Feminist Practice and Post-structuralist Theory*, Oxford: Basil Blackwell.

White, M. (1988) 'Language and anorexia', paper presented to the Anorexia Bulima Nervosa Association, Eastern Community Health Centre, Adelaide, South Australia.

White, M. and Epston, D. (1989) *Literate Means to Therapeutic Ends*, Adelaide: Dulwich Centre Publishing.

Part IV

Governmentality

Chapter 9

Of health and statecraft

Thomas Osborne

Foucault's work is probably of very little direct use to health policy. He offers no positive conceptions as to how health might be regulated, only historical studies relating to how systems of knowledge concerning the health of populations came to be linked to styles of power and procedures of state. We should not, however, immediately despair.

FOUCAULT AND 'REACTIVE' CONCEPTIONS OF HEALTH POLICY

If Foucault is in no position to enlighten us about the current state of health policy, then this may be because he has rather a singular notion of what such 'enlightenment' might mean. In one of his last pieces, Foucault wrote of enlightenment as providing not positive blueprints for the future but the constant possibility of a kind of *Ausgang* or 'way out' (Foucault 1984). And maybe this is how Foucault should be used; as a means of exit rather than as the source of a new paradigm of enquiry.

But exit from what? Most analyses of health policy appear to adopt a *reactive* conception of the relation between health and policy. That is, on the one hand, policy is viewed as a reaction to objective problems of health need and provision, and on the other, the state of health is viewed as a product of the relative effectiveness of policy. Three broad kinds of reactive account may be distinguished; and Foucault's work may be used as a starting point for a possible way out from all of these, and maybe – as we shall see later – towards a somewhat different organisation of our *expectations* as to what health policy is and what can be done with it.

First, the *meliorist approach* considers the development of health policy in terms of the progressive adequacy of health knowledge and provision. As knowledge progresses, certain intolerabilities (diseases, obstacles to knowledge, limitations in provision) are overcome, giving rise to new health problems and challenges. Thus health policy is viewed as an evolution in relation to objective problems cropping up in the social, vital or political environment.

Far more common these days is what can be called the *critical* approach. Critical analyses of health policy have tended to introduce a certain historicism into their procedings. Here, policy is not just a reaction to objective intolerabilities, but the product of negotiations or clashes of interest between different concerned parties, interest groups or classes. But critical accounts are still reactive in so far as they attempt to measure the distance between the negotiated provision of policy and the actual problems that exist on the ground. One might cite various Marxist histories of health policy in this regard; here, policy is typically seen as the – usually inadequate – outcome of negotiations between different interest-groups in the light of certain agreed intolerabilities.

Foucault's use-value in relation to all this is not, perhaps, what has often been thought. Quite often, Foucault is mobilised under the banner of an *anti-medical approach*. This kind of perspective usually involves the claim that no such thing as an objective kind of intolerability exists; that health policy constructs its concerns, and that health problems are always relative to particular societies and contexts. Typically, however, this kind of approach tends only to replace the dualisms of reactive accounts of health policy with a monism centred on 'power', or 'desire' or some other such concept; with the result that medicine appears to colonise the social field in a negative way. A good example of this would be David Armstrong's use of Foucault in his book, *Political Anatomy of the Body* (1983); an approach which might be described as a kind of radical constructionism.

PROBLEMATISATION AND GOVERNMENTALITY

It might, however, be useful to substitute the notion of problematisation for that of constructionism. Instead of saying that issues of health policy are simply constructs (constructs of what? of power?), it can be said that such issues are always the product of particular problematisations (Foucault 1988b). Problematisations are not modes of constructing problems but active ways of positing and experiencing them. It is not that there is nothing 'out there' but constructions but that policy cannot get to work without first problematising its territory. And if this means that policy is fundamentally a creative rather than a reactive endeavour, it also means that policy can never just be about anything (as often appears to be the case with the more insistent forms of constructionism). On the contrary, the function of problematisations is to reduce complexity, to provide a field of delimitation regulating what can and cannot be said.

Foucault tied this notion of problematisation not to some abstract conception of power but especially to what he called arts of government (Foucault 1989). Such arts, he writes, function to question what he called 'the conduct of conduct'. That is, government does not just specify the subjects of government as being agents passive before power but as monads of conduct, whose conduct can be shaped in various ways and directions. Government, in other words, always tends to problematise – to put into question – the relation between those who are governed and those who govern; problematisations of government are also questionings of the very objects, means and ends of government (Foucault 1989: 99–104). This is not quite the same as a constructionist approach. For instance, as Foucault contended, the perspective of government is concerned not to show that power 'produced lunatics, criminals, or sick people where there were none, but that the various and particular forms of "government" of individuals have played a determining role in the different modes of objectification of the subject' (Foucault 1988a: 15). This means that government is never just either the effect of ideology or an unmediated reaction to events or social pressures. But nor is it merely a question of the more or less passive execution of power over others. On the contrary, to govern, in Foucault's sense, is to presuppose freedom if not necessarily as a resource then certainly as a constitutive problem for government (Burchell et al. 1991: 5, 119).

In accounts of governmentality, intelligibility not exhaustiveness is the key (Cousins and Hussain 1984: 4). What is sought is not an exhaustiveness of evidence but an intelligibility of problematisations; hence, what counts as adequate 'evidence' tends to differ here from reactive accounts of 'policy'. As will the typical objects of evidence. Instead of the usual concerns with the holy trinity of profession, state and legislation, there appears a focus on the constitution of authority over particular problem areas; in this case, various aspects of health. Authority – whether it resides in the professions, the state or law – is never just given or constructed in the abstract but always problematised, negotiated and constituted. So, for example, it might be preferable not to talk about the state as such but about something like *statecraft*, a means of, so to speak, stylising the relations between the state and the space of government; not to talk about the given interests of the professions but about the constitution of professional authority; and not to talk about legislation so much as the establishment of norms and styles of governing of which law is at most just a part, at best merely an expression.

This is not exactly a sociological approach. Sociology tends to be drawn to the analysis of institutions. Governmentality, on the other hand, concerns itself with practices not institutions. What are practices? The mistake is to view them as 'applications' of policy or ideology. Rather, practices, in this vocabulary, relate to a zone or space of governmental intervention. To focus on practices is not to focus on the hard edge of (to adopt a superannuated vocabulary) the 'real-concrete', but upon the leading edges of governmental problematisation. Collections of practices constitute mentalities of governmental reasoning. One way of capturing the essence of this approach is to observe its relative distance from the sociological level of analysis of 'the unintended consequences of action'. Rather the aim is to concentrate upon something like the 'intended consequences of action' (Hirschman 1977); that is, to concentrate upon that level of action upon which we seek to act – precisely at the level of critique, of judgement, of policy itself.

GOVERNMENTALITY AND HEALTH POLICY

How might all this relate specifically to medicine and to health policy? To answer this, we might consider some substantive themes that can be linked to this question of the relation between the pursuit of health and mentalities of government. These themes are themselves intended to be part of a problematisation – and relativisation – of what health policy might mean to us in the present.

Theme of population

In the early modern period, the arts of government first took on a secularised form. For the first time, a notion of an autonomous reason of state emerged; that is, a form of reason that directed itself to securing the greatest possible strength of the state (Foucault 1989). Hence the notion that the state has its own reasons that are proper to itself; that when one governs, one does not do so (as for instance in Machiavelli) in the interests of the Prince but in the interests of what one cares to *know* about the state itself. It is as if the territory and occupants of the state take on a kind of autonomous value. It is as if the state takes on the mantle previously held by theocratic power; the state becomes both the means and ends of government (Meinecke 1962).

Simultaneously with this novel political rationality of the state there emerged the question of the population. This concern was a novel problematisation of the linkage between ruler and the ruled; again, compare Machiavelli, for whom the function of the Prince was to retain not a population but a city-territory. But increasingly, from the early modern period, the population came to take on a positive value in its own right. The great medical historian George Rosen writes, in this context, of the emergence 'of the great Leviathan, the modern state, whose outlines slowly appear out of the storm seas of politics like a whale coming to the surface' (Rosen 1958: 86). Rosen sums up the related early modern policy of mercantilism in these terms:

> The welfare of society was regarded as identical with the welfare of the state. Since power was considered the first interest of the state, most elements of mercantilist policy were advanced and justified as strengthening the power of the realm. *Raison d'état* was the fulcrum of social policy. For policy-makers in all countries, whether in kingdoms or city-states, the important question was: What course must the government pursue to increase the national power and wealth? As the rulers and their advisers saw it, what was required was first of all a large population: second, that the population be provided for in a material sense; and thirdly, that it should be under the control of government so that it could be turned to whatever use pubic policy required.
>
> (1958: 87)

Sometimes such mercantilist doctrines became tied to the science of *police* (*polizeiwissenschaft*) – from which our notion of 'policy' derives. Here, the health of the population was a primary concern, as in the designation 'medical police'; as found for instance in the title of a work by J.P. Frank, *System einer vollstandigen medicinischen Polizey* of 1779. The Germans sought to oblige their citizenry into health. According to the linked doctrine of cameralism, the population – its health, wealth and longevity – becomes the greatest resource of the power of the state (Rosen 1953). One cannot speak of a policy specifically directed to 'health' here as such; rather police – and medical police specifically – focused upon a whole range of variables that would need regulation in pursuit of the health of the state. Policy here means those actions one takes to augment a population and its productivity in the state. Health policy, here, was not really distinct from policy *per se*. This is because in a sense all policy is related to health, in so far as the health of a population is considered a value. Policy is successful in so far as it augments the population. That is what policy is for; it designates the ideal of maximising what might be called the quantitative power of the state. Yet this ideal of medical police remained precisely that; an ideal, even if it did influence the practice of subsequent German public health – above all, determining its characteristically 'forensic' character (Macleod 1968: 204).

Theme of a right to health

From the idea that it is the duty of a government to secure the well-being of a population, it is not such a large step – and a nice instance, besides, of the strategic 'reversability' of power relations – to the parallel idea that it is a right of the population to be provided with health and well-being. In what amounts to an interesting experiment in the history of health policy, the French revolutionaries sought to implement a 'right' to health. One historian, La Berge, writes that:

> Before and during the Revolution, French reforming physicians incorporated the social contract idea into their theory of public health. The Health Committee of the National Constituent Assembly formally supported the claim that health was a natural right to which all citizens were entitled and asserted that if governments were instituted to protect natural rights, then public health was the duty of the state.
>
> (La Berge 1992: 16; cf. Weiner 1993: 5–6, 318–19)

In fact, the German idea of medical police and the French ideal of a right to health for all have a certain amount in common in that they both assume a one-way, *determinate* relationship between statecraft and the production of health. They take this to mean different things. The Germans want a kind of state espionage to institute a universal health, and the French want health to be something that can be had on demand from the state. In the one, the pursuit of health is an aspect of statecraft. In the other, statecraft is an aspect of the pursuit of health. In each, the relation can be described as being determinate in that the augmentation of one value (health or statecraft) will result in the augmentation of the other. The modernity of health policy, however, emerged when a gap opened up between the two terms of health and policy; when the relation between them was implicitly acknowledged to be dogged by a certain indeterminacy.

THE ESSENTIAL INDETERMINACY OF HEALTH POLICY

Now the problem with these ideas about health and statecraft is that – as the French found out – it is simply impossible to institute a determinate 'right' to health. There is an apparantly banal – but none the less fundamental – reason for this; to the effect that health, to have any meaning, must be posited as a biological concept, outside of the remit of any direct policy. That is, health must be, at least in part, a matter of fate. 'Health – good health – cannot derive from a right; good and bad health, however crude or subtle the criteria used, are facts; physical states and mental states' (Foucault 1988c: 170). This is not to say that there can be no such thing as health policy, but only that health cannot be a direct aspect of citizenship, but only an *indirect* one. That is, governments can at best provide the conditions – a medical staffing of the population, a hospital system, procedures of public health, sanitary infrastructures, social security, employment legislation, etc. – that put different sectors of the population on a more or less equal footing with regard to chances for health; and they can pay professionals to attempt to cure (where possible) diseases after they have occurred. But they cannot guarantee health as such.

But there is also a further, if related, dimension to this question of the unrealisability of health policy. That remarkable philosopher of biology and medicine, Georges Canguilhem, once remarked (glossing René Leriche) that health was 'life lived in the silence of the organs'. In other words, health is essentially a negative state rather than a positive one; when one is healthy one is oblivious of the issue of health or ill-health as a problem (Canguilhem 1989). Health, in this sense, is something we cannot know positively; or at least we can only know it, so to speak, in its absence. Canguilhem argues further that health is not designated by anything that can be defined as the 'normal' but by normativity – that is, the capacity to institute new norms upon one's environment. 'Man feels in good health – which is health itself – only when he feels more than normal – that is, adapted to the environment and its demands – but normative, capable of following new norms of life' (Canguilhem 1989: 200).

In other words, health is not an absolute or determinate concept but an essentially indeterminate, relative or elastic one. It is possible to institute measures designed to ward off preventable sicknesses, one can institute measures designed to cure existing ills, but in the process – even if one eradicates all known diseases – one will not have instituted an absolute ideal called 'health'. This is because with every act of provision the very sphere of what constitutes health will begin to widen and extend, until even death – or perhaps even life itself – becomes a perceived form of ill-health. This has an important consequence. It means that one can never have a style of government of which the end is simply 'health'. As Albert Hirschman says when discussing mechanisms of disappointment, what were once positive pleasures soon become just comforts or necessities – and he might have been thinking of all that more or less taken-for-granted apparatus of our health provision today; sewage systems, drinking water, basic medical facilities and so on. These are forms of provision that were once an aspect of *health* policy but which have now become the technical objects of social or environmental policy (Hirschman 1982: 27, quoted in Jacob 1988: 71). In other words, each time government takes steps towards the target of 'health' the thing itself escapes over the horizon, leaving behind only technical problems and arguments over resources. As Foucault himself succinctly glosses this issue: 'The problem raised is, therefore, that of the relationship between an infinite demand and a finite system' (Foucault 1988a: 173).

It needs to be emphasised that to invoke the essential elasticity or indeterminacy of the concept of health in relation to policy is not necessarily – as it has been, on occasion, for those on the Right – a recipe for retrenchment in the field of health policy. The consequences may not be so drastic. This indeterminacy is rather something we have to live with – even defend. For this elasticity is only expressive of the fact that health cannot be associated with normality but only with normativity, with the capacity to impose new norms. Health, in other words, necessarily escapes the activities of health policy – otherwise we cannot even speak of health in a meaningful way at all.

Indeed, one has only to consider the political consequences of attempts to absolutise – to make determinate – the concept of health, to see the pertinence of this. It often seems as if such initiatives tend in the direction – putting it contentiously – of a *polizeiwissenschaft* of health; 'policy' reverts to its root, *police*. And if, indeed, one thinks of those kinds of regime that have attempted to make health a goal of political ideals, it is difficult to resist a certain pressure to shudder inwardly. One moves very quickly from the idea of health being a right of citizenship to that of health being a duty of citizenship. The aspirations in this area of such diverse ideological formations as the political culture of Nazism and the well-intentioned programmes of the proponents of the Peckham (Pioneer) Health Centre in Britain, in this sense at least, have something in common – the temptation to turn health into an absolute concept and hence a kind of duty; and – as if the consequences needed spelling out – ill-health, disease, disability, difference as a kind of failing, deviation or sin. Such totalising procedures, instead of instituting health, seem only to corrupt the very notion of health. They substitute for a certain 'concern for normativity' the project of a normalising imposition of norms. In these cases, we cannot speak of health as such – or of a health policy that would be a normalisation *in the name* of normativity – but only of, so to speak, a normalisation in the name of the norm.

Now, what are the consequences of these remarks for the idea of health policy as we know it? If health policy is to embody a concern for the normativity of life, then it will have to acknowledge, surely, a certain *modesty* of approach. This entails, at once, a certain respect for the necessarily mediate or *technological* aspect of health policy. Rather than seeing the history of health policy in the form of a single continuum, it might be preferable to focus on diverse technologies of health; that is, all the diverse means, projects and devices through which the impossible dream of a healthy population has been made an object of realisation. This would not be a question of deconstructing health policy and then giving up on the matter, but of conducting a kind of historical fieldwork of problematisations in technologies of health; and a question, perhaps, of attempting to tie such technologies to wider political rationalities of government.

There have been (at least) two kinds of rationality of health policy that are relevant here; that is, which have attempted to problematise the essentially indeterminate character of health policies. The one seeks out a sort of naturalism of health; the other seeks out a sort of constructivism of it. A *liberal* government of health, it could be said, does not seek to act directly upon health itself, but only indirectly, in the form of imposing techniques of security levied on the environment (Gordon 1991). A *neo-liberal* government acts directly upon health by giving the ideal of health a series of surrogate values, entailing a sort of constructivism of goals and targets intended to bring about strategically limited objectives. But, in the end, these alternatives are just different ways of conceptualising what we have designated as the inherently 'technological' aspect of health policy; the one seeks out what could be called indirect technologies, the other seeks out direct, strategic technologies but related only to limited objectives. In what follows, we are restricted to some more or less schematic remarks relating to this distinction.

It is worth stressing that the discussion that follows is a rather generalised one; and that the designations of liberalism and neo-liberalism are more like abstract logics or heuristic diagrams of policy than empirically observable expressions of events. Liberalism and neo-liberalism, in this specific usage, are best seen as concepts with which to measure reality rather than as realities upon which we should go about building concepts.

LIBERALISM AND NEO-LIBERALISM

In *The Conflict of the Faculties* (1979), Kant asked himself, amongst other things – what sort of a discipline is medicine? Kant's text is really a reflection on the proper limits of government in relation to the spheres of truth, law and health. Over the sphere of law (and, in a different way, theology), which is a public discipline, Kant says, government should have a controlling discretion; and over philosophy – given that philosophy is concerned with the disinterested establishment of truth – government should refrain from intervention altogether. But what of medicine? After all, health is a matter for government in so far as the health of the population is a concern of the state; yet, the provision of health is also related to the pursuit of truth – concerning the norms of population and the body – and, as such, should be a matter of political indifference on the part of government. Kant's solution is effectively to say that medicine is a kind of intermediate technology, existing between the sphere of the state and the disinterestedness of truth; a kind of hybrid discipline, existing between the demands of truth and government. What the state must do is not to dictate the norms of health in the interests of government, but to regulate the production of truth by governing not health itself but those who are delegated to speak in the name of health, that is, the medical profession.

A crude formula for this might be that liberal forms of government direct health policy always at a certain distance or remove. They embrace the indeterminate character of health policy. They seek to bring about health as a kind of deliberately intended by-product of their activities. A liberal capacity to govern will tend to stress the provision of infrastructural conditions of healthy living – sewage systems, clean water-supply, a state-regulated but not state-controlled medical profession – but at the expense, in the main, of direct injunctions to lead a healthy lifestyle, to transform oneself in the interests of one's own health and longevity (Osborne 1996). Of course, it may be up to the medical profession to perform these kinds of functions relating to the education of persons with regard to their own health. The point is only that such a demand is not inscribed within the political rationality of liberal government itself; for the most part, the role of statecraft is to regulate infrastructures – to provide what Foucault terms, in this context, 'apparatuses of security' (Gordon 1991: 19–21) – and to delegate powers of health to an accredited medical profession. In this latter context, we can indeed talk about a 'liberal' profession of medicine; not in the sense of the old pre-modern 'liberal professions' but in the sense of a liberal art of government that legitimates a medical profession in the interests of an indirect government of health (Osborne 1993).

It should be emphasised at this point that liberalism here does not refer to anything like party-political allegiance – and still less to any philosophical doctrine – but rather to a way of problematising the question of government. One way to think about liberalism is in terms of a crisis of 'reason of state'. For the liberal thinkers of the nineteenth century, it became increasingly clear that the actions of the state could actually serve to frustrate the ends of the state itself; too much intervention led to a distortion of the territory to be governed (Foucault 1989; Barry *et al.* 1996). But liberalism is not simply about the absence of the state, or policies of laissez-faire. The liberal notion of population is critical here, and can provide a heuristic contrast with notions of population in police and cameralism. The liberal conception of population is as a natural domain; there are 'processes of population' that are integral to themselves, that is, which are conceived as being autonomous and which require not directive intervention but delicate sustenance on the part of government through apparatuses of security and arts of knowledge such as the disciplines of political economy, statistics and public health (Gordon 1991).

This relative impermeability of processes of population is significant for liberal government in that such processes become, as it were, 'test-beds' with regard to the probity of the state and the efficacy of government itself (Foucault 1989: 109–10). This can be illustrated by recourse to a distinction between styles of health policy in Britain and France in the nineteenth century. Whereas, as Foucault puts it, in France medicine began with a war on bad government (meaning that medicine was an aspect of government itself, and that the doctor was a legislator), in Britain, where doctors were never to be allowed to aspire to be legislators, ill-health quickly became an indicator or signal of bad government (Foucault 1973: 33, 1989: 110). In short, with regard to Britain, the alternative to viewing the history of health policy according to any of the reactive variants is not a thesis of medicalisation, but actually something like the opposite – entailing an exploration of the varied ways in which the function of the state was problematised with regard to the health of subjects. Indeed, as a general though not particularly revealing hypothesis, one might say that far from being a medicalisation of Europe, what was at stake in the nineteenth century was a mode of governing health that owed something to liberalism.

None of this is to say that liberal government was particularly coherent, successful or unresisted. Indeed, there is a logic to the resistance that it generated. Above all, the problem relates to what might or might not count as an indirect technology of health. What are the limits to what is required? What is the proper responsibility of government in relation to these limits? For instance, a very prominent theme of resistance to liberal conceptions of health policy is that they entail too limited a notion of what counts as a strategy of security. It is characteristic of liberalism to emphasise the delegation of health functions to a (curative) medical profession; direct measures of prevention (health campaigns, health education and so forth) are typically held in some suspicion as an over-extension of the remit of government. Yet, in opposition to this, critics have consistently argued that such proactive campaigns should also be counted as aspects of security.

In this context, so-called 'socialised' versions of health policy should not be seen as being in radical discontinuity with liberal strategies for the government of health. Socialised medicine – at least in the capitalist countries – has typically been, rather, a question of an expansion of what counts as a regime of security. The British National Health Service, for example, was established as a homogenisation and rationalisation of the existing system of medical care rather than as a new beginning along wholly new principles (Webster 1988). Moreover, the style of medicine promoted in the service has always leaned very heavily towards a delegation of curative functions rather than a proactive provision of preventive functions; and considerable autonomy has been allowed to practitioners of all kinds in the service. However, socialised medicine of this kind pushes the logic of liberal health policy to its limit in so far as it tends towards a system whereby government actually takes responsibility for the health of its citizens. Foucault himself clearly regarded the establishment of the service in these terms; that is, as something of a 'break' in systems of health policy; 'Just at the moment when war was causing wholesale destruction, a society took upon itself the task of explicitly guaranteeing to its members not only the fact of life, but also a life lived in good health' (Foucault 1994: 40). As such, no doubt, it could be said that the logic of a socialised health policy leads in either of two directions; either *beyond* liberalism towards a properly socialised – that is, something like a social*ist* – service; or – as seems to have been the case in Britain and in most of the English-speaking countries since the 1980s – *away* from liberalism and in the direction of something like a neo-liberal government of health.

Even so, the logic of neo-liberalism embarks from the same point as that of liberalism itself. It departs from the same problem but, as it were, problematises it differently. Each begins from a certain implicit recognition of the essential indeterminacy of health policy. Unlike liberalism, however, which posits immanent processes of population and modulated apparatuses of security, neo-liberalism proposes what can be described as a governmental constructivism (Burchell 1996: 27–30). In other words, whereas liberalism proposed indirect technologies to bring about health as a kind of by-product, neo-liberalism, in proposing to make technologies of health as 'direct' as possible, is fundamentally a strategic rather than a naturalistic governmental rationality. Neo-liberalism proposes 'surrogate' variables that will stand measure for otherwise abstract ideas of health; above all, in the form of targets relating to finance, pharmaceuticals, recovery rates, operations, patients, waiting-lists and so forth – tending even towards a generalised quantification of the health field. In short, in response to the indeterminacy of health policy, neo-liberalism constructs the possibility of its strictly de-limited determination.

Neo-liberalism abandons the quest for an absolute that would be 'health' and opts for determinant strategies, targets and specifics instead. Hence two phenomena which are most characteristic of neo-liberal versions of health policy: first, that language which is very typical of the neo-liberal mentality, centred on the strict specification of de-limited and targeted domains for intervention. To take one well-known example from the field of public health in Britain, the document *The Health of the Nation*; this involved the establishment of prevention targets in five de-limited areas; heart disease and strokes, cancers, mental illness, sexual health and accidents, and lifestyle-associated conditions. This kind of strategic approach is really only the complement of a whole series of technologies designed to instrumenta-lise health policy – league tables, audit measures, clinical trials, Quality Adjusted Life Years (QALYs) and so forth.

The second phenomenon is the imposition of an immanent principle of functioning intended to operate throughout the whole system and intended to animate and regulate it; namely, that of 'responsibilisation'. It is not only, as some critics have noted, that people are made responsible for their own health; with all the 'victim-blaming' consequences this implies. Rather, the principle of reponsibilisation works like a moving force throughout the whole system, giving it coherence as its principle of functioning. So managers are to be responsible for managing hospitals as businesses, general practitioners are to be responsible for managing and budgeting their practices, and patients and, of course, potential patients are to be responsible for being entrepreneurs of their own health. Because health is not an absolute value, neo-liberalism attempts to construct values according to a kind of immanent logic – it involves a kind of boot-strapping of surrogate health-values; targets are set, market-exchanges take place, performance is monitored, success and failure rates are measured, new targets are set, further market-exchanges take place. . . .

CONCLUSION

The problem, anyway, is not really with the 'failure' of health policy. In fact, health policy just has to fail. Perhaps that is the most obvious conclusion that can be drawn from our attempt to put some of Foucault's and Canguilhem's concepts to work in relation to this field. This does not mean, however, that we are powerless to act. But it may mean that we need to be careful about how we address our criticisms to dominant strands of health policy. For instance, criticisms of the logic of neo-liberalism have been very widespread. Rather than address these criticisms in depth here, just two comments can be made. First, it would be a mistake to regard the neo-liberal approach to health policy as being the exclusive property of the Right (even if in most countries this so far has, in fact, been the case). Rather, one of the features of neo-liberalism has been its propensity – as with the Healthy Cities movement and the 'new public health', for example – to forge alliances and alignments across the political spectrum.

The second point is merely to observe that criticisms of neo-liberal health policy from the perspective of the Left often fail to acknowledge the coherence, or at least the inventiveness, of neo-liberalism as well as the fact that neo-liberal health policy begins not merely from a malign desire to roll back the state and renege on funding commitments but from what is actually a more or less legitimate or, at least, coherent problematisation of the situation of health policy – namely, the fact that there cannot meaningfully be such a thing as an absolute 'right' to health. Perhaps, in the end, the only sure way of assessing the value of a system of health provision lies in gauging whether or not such a system rolls back, in Hirschman's sense, the direction of the movement from pleasures to comforts or necessities. If it can be shown – which indeed in some cases, and certainly in the case of Britain, it can – that neo-liberal policies have made goods that had become necessities once again a matter only of pleasure (and indeed privilege) then it can surely be said that the fortunes of health policy have indeed suffered something like a reversal. In such a situation, we have something like a health policy which lumbers towards a condition of what Foucault would have called 'intolerability'.

And is there a 'way out' of the generic impossibility of health policy? Perhaps the only sure way out is to exit from an exclusive attention to health as a value in policy terms in the first place. In Britain, it has been a common response to the Black Report, which in the early 1980s exposed widespread and fundamental inequalities in health, to argue that the real solution to inequalities in ill-health involves reference to features that might be seen as properly belonging outside of the health sphere as narrowly defined; that is, in the domain of housing, social welfare and the provision of utilities (Davey Smith *et al.* 1990). In this sense, a focus on health as such might be seen as something of a diversion; and the war against ill-health might indeed be conceived, as Foucault said of the French revolutionaries, rather as 'a war against bad government'. Perhaps the notion of policy specifically directed towards a population's health as a value in its own right has, in this sense, merely been a long diversion. The point might be – still – to change society.

REFERENCES

Armstrong, D. (1983) *Political Anatomy of the Body*, Cambridge: Cambridge University Press.

Barry, A., Osborne, T. and Rose, N. (eds) (1996) *Foucault and Political Reason*, London: University College London Press.

Burchell, G. (1996) 'Liberal government and techniques of the self', in A. Barry, T. Osborne and N. Rose (eds) *Foucault and Political Reason*, London: University College London Press.

Burchell, G., Gordon, C. and Miller, P. (1991) *The Foucault Effect*, Hemel Hempstead: Harvester-Wheatsheaf.

Canguilhem, G. (1989) *The Normal and the Pathological*, trans. C. Fawcett, Dordrecht: Reidel.

Cousins, M. and Hussain, A. (1984) *Michel Foucault*, London: Macmillan.

Davey Smith, G., Bartley, M. and Blane, D. (1990) 'The Black Report on socioeconomic inequalities in health ten years on', *British Medical Journal*, 301, 18–25 August: 373–7.

Foucault, M. (1973) *The Birth of the Clinic*, trans. A. Sheridan-Smith, London: Tavistock.

Foucault, M. (1984) 'What is Enlightenment?', in P. Rabinow (ed.) *The Foucault Reader*, Harmondsworth: Pelican.

Foucault, M. (M. Florence) (1988a) '(Auto-)biography', *History of the Present*, 4 (Spring): 13–15.

Foucault, M. (1988b) 'On problematization', *History of the Present*, 4 (Spring): 16–17.

Foucault, M. (1988c) 'Social security', in L. Kritzman (ed.) *Michel Foucault: Politics, Philosophy, Culture*, London: Routledge.

Foucault, M. (1989) *Resumé des cours*, Paris: Juillard.

Foucault, M. (1994) 'Crise de la médicine ou crise de l'antimédicine', in *Dits et Ecrits*, volume III, pp. 40–58, Paris: Gallimard.

Gordon, C. (1991) 'Governmentality – an introduction', in G. Burchell, C. Gordon and P. Miller (eds) *The Foucault Effect*, Hemel Hempstead: Harvester-Wheatsheaf.

Hirschman, A. (1977) *The Passions and the Interests*, Princeton: Princeton University Press.

Hirschman, A. (1982) *Shifting Involvements*, Princeton: Princeton University Press.

Jacob, J. (1988) *Doctors and Rules*, London: Routledge.

Kant, I. (1979) *The Conflict of the Faculties*, trans. M.J. Gregor, Lincoln, Nebraska: University of Nebraska Press.

la Berge, A. (1992) *Mission and Method*, Cambridge: Cambridge University Press.

Macleod, R. (1968) 'The anatomy of state medicine: concept and application', in F.N.L. Poynter (ed.) *Medicine and Science in the 1860s*, London: Wellcome Institute.

Meinecke, F. (1962) *Machiavellism: The Doctrine of Reason of State and its Place in Modern History*, trans. D. Scott, London: Routledge and Kegan Paul.

Osborne, T. (1993) 'On liberalism, neo-liberalism and the "liberal profession" of medicine', *Economy and Society*, 22, 3: 345–56.

Osborne, T. (1996) 'Security and vitality: drains, liberalism and power in the nineteenth century', in A. Barry, T. Osborne and N. Rose (eds) *Foucault and Political Reason*, London: University College London Press.

Rosen, G. (1953) 'Cameralism and the concept of medical police', *Bulletin of Historical Medicine*, 27: 21–42.

Rosen, G. (1958) *A History of Public Health*, Cambridge, Massachusetts: Harvard University Press.

Webster, C. (1988) *The Health Services Since the War*, volume 1, London: HMSO.

Weiner, D. (1993) *The Citizen-Patient in Revolutionary and Imperial Paris*, Baltimore: Johns Hopkins University Press.

Chapter 10

Risk, governance and the new public health

Alan Petersen

This chapter explores the utility of the concepts of risk and governance, as developed by Foucauldian scholars, in the analysis of the health promotion strategies of the so-called new public health. It begins by examining some problems and limitations with the influential, and conventional modernist, perspectives on risk and the self proposed by Ulrich Beck and Anthony Giddens, before moving on to examine an approach, suggested particularly in the work of Robert Castel, which analyses risk and prevention as aspects of contemporary techniques of governance. Castel's view is that in many contemporary 'neo-liberal' societies there has been a broad shift in forms of surveillance and control from those based upon the direct, face-to-face relationship between experts and subjects to those based upon the abstract calculation of risk. The chapter shows how this development has been manifested in a number of recent health promotion strategies of the new public health, and then concludes with a discussion of some implications of the governmentality concept for the further analysis of the new public health.

THE CONCEPT OF RISK IN SOCIOLOGY

The concept of risk has come to assume increasing prominence in sociological writings on late modern society, witnessed by the proliferation of socio-cultural analyses of risk and of studies which have explored the implications of a new risk consciousness for personal conduct (e.g. Beck 1992, 1995; Castel 1991; Douglas 1990, 1992; Douglas and Wildavsky 1982; Giddens 1991; Luhmann 1993). Although recent literature reflects a diverse range of perspectives on risk, it is the work of Ulrich Beck and Anthony Giddens that has come to dominate recent sociological thinking in this area. Beck and Giddens share a number of key assumptions about modernity and subjectivity that are profoundly questioned by Foucault's post-structuralism. Both writers have explored the implications of the new risk climate, characterised by the existence of 'high-consequence risks' linked to processes of industrialisation and globalisation, for the self-creation of identity and a personal sense of security. In a context of heightened concerns about global environmental crisis, the work of both writers would seem to have found a ready audience among those seeking to make some sense of the global context of risk and establish some basis for personal decision-making in the face of apparent increasing uncertainty. Despite some differences in their theoretical schemas and use of terminology, both Beck and Giddens see 'risk' as central to late modern culture, and as having become a key element in the calculations of the self. (For a discussion of differences and similarities in Beck's and Giddens's work see Beck *et al.* 1994 and Lash and Urry 1994: 31–59.)

Clearly, Beck and Giddens have contributed substantially to the development of a new paradigm for sociological research on risk. However, the work of each can be seen to have considerable problems and limitations, linked largely to their adherence to conventional modernist views on self, science and society. Both can be criticised for their lack of attention to the aesthetic-expressive dimension of the modern self, the lack of acknowledgement of the 'embodied' nature of the self, and a cognitive bias in their idea of reflexivity whereby the body is an object to be monitored by the ego or subject (Lash and Urry 1994: 38–46). Giddens in particular has been criticised for adopting a positivist ego psychology which is hostile to any notion that the self is complexly structured and differentiated (Lash and Urry 1994: 42). Moreover, as Lash notes, neither theorist offers an effective critique of expertise in his proposals for alternative and democratic institutions, which are seen to involve the lay public 'voting' on competing forms of expertise and provide little room for the 'participatory democracy' of informal everyday politics and social movements (Lash 1994: 201). Beck sees science as both a cause of and the source of solutions to risks. However, science's potential to solve problems is seen as compromised by its subordination to bureaucratic and industrial imperatives such that it no longer operates 'in the service of truth' (1992: 166). In Beck's view, science can change itself and elevate the inherent reflexivity of the modernisation process into its forms of thought and work so that reason can be activated and mobilised against uncertainty (1992: 179–81; see also Beck 1995: 111–27). The subject of Beck's and Giddens's accounts is an autonomous rational ego who uses expert systems reflexively to regulate everyday life. For Giddens, these expert systems are quintessentially social-scientific knowledge and techniques of self-therapy; for Beck, they are the spread of lay knowledges in regard to science and the environment (Lash and Urry 1994: 54). In the work of neither writer is the concept of the autonomous rational actor of modernist discourse opened to critical scrutiny. Their notion of reflexivity is bound up with an orthodox conception of modernity and modernisation which is underpinned by a meta-narrative of progress and evolving self-consciousness. When modernisation reaches a certain level, agents become 'individualised', that is, less constrained by structures, and the self becomes a project to be reflexively fashioned.

According to Giddens, in the post-traditional society, the self undergoes massive change since the constraints over choice are effectively weakened, and the individual is confronted with a complex diversity of alternatives, especially in relation to 'lifestyle'. All elements of 'life-planning', such as decisions about relationships and careers, involve complex issues of choice, of preparing a course of future actions, which are mobilised in terms of the self's biography (Giddens 1991: 80–7). Giddens sees trust in others and in abstract systems as crucial to the reflexive fashioning of the self. Trust established between the infant and its caretakers allows the individual to develop a sense of ontological security, and trust in abstract systems (e.g. the monetary system, expertise) is necessary if the individual is to avoid becoming paralysed by anxieties. The more tradition loses its hold, and daily life is reconstituted in terms of the relationship between the local and the global, the more reflexively organised life-planning involves trust in others, especially experts. Living in a climate of global risk, however, is 'inherently unsettling' for the individual, especially given the scope and intensity of global transformations which influence the very constitution of the self, and so feelings of anxiety and 'crisis' become an endemic, 'normal' part of the individual's experience (1991: 181–5).

For Beck, too, once the individual is 'cut loose' from traditional commitments and support relationships, he or she must choose between a diverse array of lifestyles, subcultures, social ties and identities. 'Class' and the nuclear family no longer determine one's personal outlook, lifestyles, ideologies and identities. This is not to say that 'class' and family cease to have any significance at all, or that individuality is unconstrained. Rather, it is Beck's view that individuality in late modern society is largely played out within the constraints of 'secondary agencies and institutions', principally the labour market, and in the arena of consumption. These agencies and institutions create their own kinds of dependency: upon fashions, social policy, and economic cycles and markets. Individuals must learn, 'on pain of permanent disadvantage', to conceive of themselves as the masters of their own fate, and to see events and conditions that happen to them to be a consequence of their own decisions. Like Giddens, Beck sees the individual as actively engaged in shaping his or her own biography and making decisions according to calculations of risk and opportunity. One chooses one's identity and group membership, and in the process partakes in the individualisation of risks. Whereas what assails the individual was previously considered a 'blow of fate' sent by God or nature (e.g. war, natural catastrophes, death of a spouse), it is now much more likely to be events that are considered a 'personal failure', such as not passing an examination, unemployment or divorce (1992: 127–37).

The idea of the self-reflexive, autonomous subject that is evident in the analyses of Beck and Giddens, and indeed those of many other contemporary writers on modernity, is profoundly challenged by the work of Foucault and his followers. Although Foucault himself did not directly address the topic of 'risk', his writings on governmentality laid the groundwork for an analysis of risk as a political technology (see e.g. Castel 1991; Ewald 1991). The article by Robert Castel (1991: 281–98), 'From dangerousness to risk', is of particular relevance in this respect because not only does he draw attention to the role of expertise in the administration of populations and the regulation of personal identity, which are neglected dimensions in the work of both Beck and Giddens, but his analysis focuses specifically on the new preventive strategies that have emerged in a number of contemporary societies and that can be seen to be manifest in various practices of the new public health.

RISK AS GOVERNANCE

Evidently indebted to Foucault's work on 'governmentality' (see e.g. Foucault 1991), Castel has drawn attention to the emergence of new preventive strategies of social administration, evident in a number of contemporary societies, which 'dissolve the notion of the subject or a concrete individual, and put in its place a combinatory of factors, the factors of risk' (Castel 1991: 281). Castel's argument is that over the last hundred years there has been a shift in emphasis from controlling the dangerous individual, via face-to-face interventions of preventive medicine and use of confinement, to an emphasis on anticipating and preventing the emergence of undesirable events such as illness, abnormality and deviant behaviour. As Castel notes, 'a risk does not arise from the presence of particular precise danger embodied in a concrete individual or group. It is the effect of a combination of abstract *factors* which render more or less probable the occurrence of undesirable modes of behaviour' (Castel 1991: 287, emphasis in original).

This shift, argues Castel, represents the imposition of a far more subtle and effective mode of population regulation than that implied by the identification and control of aberrant individuals and multiplies the possibilities for intervention. By focusing not on individuals but on factors of risk, on statistical correlations of heterogeneous elements, the experts have multiplied the possibilities for preventive intervention. As Castel asks, 'for what situation is there for which one can be certain that it harbours no risk, no uncontrollable or unpredictable chance feature?' In the name of absolute eradication of risks, the experts have constructed a mass of new risks which constitute so many new targets for preventive intervention. Surprisingly, he says, there has been little trace of any reflection on 'the social and human costs of this new witch-hunt'; for instance, the *'iatrogenic aspects of prevention* which in fact are always operative even when it is consumption of such "suspect" products as alcohol or tobacco and alcohol which is under attack' (Castel 1991: 289, emphases in original).

Castel is not the first or only writer to point to the regulatory effects of risk and prevention in modern societies. However, unlike others, who have tended to restrict their analysis to the symbolic and rhetorical role of prevention and risk in mobilising the support of citizens in the reconstruction of social problems and/or in regulating boundaries between the Self and Other (e.g. Crawford 1994; Douglas 1990, 1992; Douglas and Wildavsky 1982; Freeman 1991), Castel examines prevention and risk in relation to the distinctive political rationalities and techniques of the contemporary period. He asks whether the emergence of new preventive strategies is part of a set of new management techniques of a kind specific to 'neo-liberal' societies. As a number of writers have recently pointed out, these are societies characterised by a form of political rationality that reactivates liberal principles: an emphasis on markets as regulators of economic activity; scepticism over the capacities of governments to properly govern; and the replacement of 'welfare dependency' by active entrepreneurship (Burchell 1993; Gordon 1991; Rose 1993; Rose and Miller 1992: 198). Castel notes that new forms of control are appearing in these societies which work not through repression or welfare interventionism, but through 'assign[ing] different social destinies to individuals in line with their varying capacity to live up to the requirements of competitiveness and profitability' (1991: 294). Any type of difference can potentially be objectified, and made a basis for assigning a special destiny to certain categories defined in this way as a matter of political will. And the development of computer technology has made this technically feasible (Castel 1991: 294–5).

Neo-liberalism is a form of rule which involves creating a sphere of freedom for subjects so that they are able to exercise a regulated autonomy. While both early liberal and neo-liberal rationalities of government have been premised upon the self-conduct of the governed themselves, neo-liberal rationality is linked to a form of rational self-conduct that is not so much a given of human nature (i.e. the interest-motivated, rational ego) as a consciously contrived style of conduct (Burchell 1993; Gordon 1991: 41–5; Rose 1993). As Rose observes, neo-liberal rationality emphasises the entrepreneurial individual, endowed with freedom and autonomy, and the capacity to properly care for him- or herself (Rose 1993: 288). Although expertise still continues to play a crucial role in government, the authority of expertise is increasingly separated from the apparatuses of political rule, and located in the market 'governed by the rationalities of competition, accountability and consumer demand' (1993: 285). The idea of one's life as the enterprise of oneself implies that 'one remains always continuously employed in (at least) that one enterprise, and that it is part of the continuous business of living to make adequate provision for the preservation, reproduction and reconstruction of one's own human capital' (Gordon 1991: 44). Neo-liberalism calls upon the individual to enter into the process of his or her own self-governance through processes of endless self-examination, self-care and self-improvement. Given that the 'care of the self' is bound up with the project of moderating the burden of individuals on society, it is not surprising that it is in the health promotion strategies of the so-called new public health that these developments are most apparent. As many commentators have noted, since the mid-1970s, there has been a clear ideological shift away from the notion that the state should protect the health of individuals to the idea that individuals should take responsibility to protect themselves from risk (e.g. Scott and Williams 1991). A close examination of the recent goals of health promotion and of its related strategies shows how the processes of risk management have, in effect, served the objective of privatising health by distributing responsibility for managing risk throughout the social body while at the same time creating new possibilities for intervention into private lives.

HEALTH PROMOTION AND THE PRODUCTION OF THE 'AT RISK' SELF

The emergence of the new public health signals a considerable broadening of the focus of health promotion which has come to take as its object the 'environment', conceived in its broadest sense, spanning the local through to the global level and including social, psychological and physical elements (see e.g. Ashton 1992; Ashton and Seymour 1988; Davies and Kelly 1993). With the emergence of this broad concept of determining environment in the new public health, the distinction between healthy and unhealthy populations totally dissolves since everything potentially is a source of 'risk' and everyone can be seen to be 'at risk'. Contemporary health promotion encompasses such areas as community development, personal skills development, the control of advertising 'unhealthy' and dangerous products, the regulation of urban space (e.g. the 'Healthy Cities' project), intervention in workplaces, and the monitoring and periodic screening of sub-populations. The encroachment of health promotion into these areas has multiplied the number of sites for preventive action, and given rise to an endless parade of 'at risk' populations and 'risky' situations. As Castel observes, all manner of interventions and prescriptions (including the demand for 'more self-care') can be deduced and justified on the basis of the calculation of the probability that an undesirable behaviour may occur and can therefore be prevented (1991: 287).

Given the scope of endeavours to identify and manage 'risks' within health promotion, it no longer makes sense to ask who exactly are the 'victims' or who is doing the 'blaming', as sociologists in the past have been inclined to do, for everyone has, in effect, become a 'victim' and, the health promoters are not clearly seen to be directly intervening, or coercing, or punishing. Health promoters indeed see themselves working at a distance through the efforts of others by way of forging collaborative ventures (e.g. 'inter-sectoral collaboration'), lobbying for policy change ('healthy public policy'), promoting community action ('community development') and making alliances with the ecology movement ('sustainable development') (Bunton 1992: 9). Contemporary health promoters have been at the forefront in the call for efforts to reorganise social institutions, and to implement different kinds and levels of intervention and collaboration involving public and private sectors, in fulfilment of the World Health Organization's goal of 'Health for All'. In their efforts to identify and control the 'factors of risk', health promoters have taken on the roles of expert mediators, programme coordinators, and 'community developers'. Health promoters are helping to forge a new conception of the political and see themselves as closely allied with the new social movements in their concern to 'empower' citizens (see e.g. Labonte 1990; Wallerstein 1993; Yeo 1993).

In Australia, the development and implementation of a series of health promotion 'goals and targets' show just how sophisticated risk profiling has become, taking into account both 'objective' determinants of health and 'subjective' measures of well-being (Commonwealth of Australia 1993: 7, 1994). The Commonwealth and State/Territory Health Ministers agreed in 1993 that the national health goals and targets ought to be embedded within the broader framework of a National Health Policy, and set in place a process for selecting initial focus areas for national agreement and action (Commonwealth of Australia 1994: 1–2). Australia, like some other countries (the US, England and Wales, and to some extent New Zealand), has in recent years developed such targets to 'guide decision-making in relation to health services provision and health promotion activities' (Commonwealth of Australia 1993: 10). In 1993, these national goals and targets were refined with the explicit aim of broadening the 'framework of action', and setting in place mechanisms for accountability and the monitoring of progress, and more fully engaging the health system in health promotion (Commonwealth of Australia 1993: 8–9). The 'extended framework' that was proposed included an elaborate schema identifying health goals and targets (including estimated date of achievable change) for a large range of 'preventable mortality and morbidity' in relation to different 'priority populations' (defined by age, gender, ethnicity, Aboriginality, socio-economic status and place of residence). It also sought to identify lifestyle and risk factors, personal knowledge and skills, and environmental determinants of health that need action in respect to each of a range of identified preventable conditions. The addition of a category focusing on personal knowledge and skills, including 'life skills' (defined as 'resilience and coping'), affirms the contemporary significance of one's life as an enterprise of oneself. To use the authors' words, 'people's ability to care for themselves, and their access to self-help and social support are recognised as important factors in the achievement and maintenance of good health' (Commonwealth of Australia 1993: 15).

The focus in recent preventive programmes on the social determinants of health behaviour and aspects of the environment deemed to be influential in bringing about change vastly extends the scope of regulatory mechanisms by calling on a diverse range of public and private agencies to monitor and shape social arrangements and individual subjectivities. So-called 'healthy public policy' is characterised by an explicit concern for health and equity in all areas of policy, including education, water, sanitation, transport systems, housing, work environments, recreation facilities and food production, and not simply those traditionally associated with health services. An important health promotion concept is that of 'intersectoral collaboration', the forging of alliances between different levels of government, private bodies, non-government organisations and community groups, to create, in effect, a multi-levelled and multi-organisational network of surveillance and regulatory practices. The task of coordinating these various groups and agencies, and of seeking to utilise their efforts and prodigious resources, has been given to the professional health promoter located in government departments of health and other state-sponsored agencies.

The complex system for monitoring and regulating populations that is indicated in the goals and targets strategy is informed, and technically facilitated, by advances in the statistical calculation of risk, employing sophisticated techniques of epidemiology. Epidemiology has become so central to the public health endeavour of identifying, reducing exposure to, or eliminating 'risks' that it has become almost synonymous with the public health enterprise itself. It has a broad agenda which makes use of vast number of practices such as case studies, quantitative analyses and laboratory experiments, and contemporary epidemiologists work closely with public policy groups and public health departments to help track risk populations and to educate all populations (Fujimura and Chou 1994: 1024).

SELF-MANAGEMENT OF RISK

An emphasis on self-management of risk and self-care has become increasingly evident in the health promotion strategies of governments as well as in the economic rationales of private companies. In the following paragraphs I describe some manifestations of this development and examine some implications for the self and for its relations with others, including experts. In particular, I point to the uncertainties generated by the subject's reliance on expertise which is increasingly located in the 'free market', where the rationalities of competition predominate.

As indicated, the notion of the individual-as-enterprise seems to have emerged as a basic premise of neo-liberal rationality. This requires the individual to adopt a calculative and prudent attitude in respect to risk and danger (Rose 1993: 296). A manifestation of this is to be found in the phenomenon of 'healthism', described by medical sociologists (Greco 1993: 357). Healthism posits that the individual has choice in preserving his or her physical capacity from the event of disease. In the event that one is unable to regulate one's own lifestyle and modify one's risky behaviour then this is, at least in part, 'a failure of the self to take care of itself' (Greco 1993: 361). Healthism has been described as 'a particular form of "bodyism" in which a hedonistic lifestyle is (paradoxically) combined with a preoccupation with ascetic practices aimed at the achievement or maintenance of appearance of health, fitness and youthfulness' (Dutton 1995: 273).

The disciplinary self-improvement demonstrated in the pursuit of health and fitness has become a key means by which individuals can express their agency and constitute themselves in conformity with the demands of a competitive world. As Crawford observes, to have a healthy body has become 'the mark of distinction that separates those who deserve to succeed from those who will fail' (1994: 1354). The terms 'healthy' and 'unhealthy' have become signifiers of normal and abnormal identity; of one's moral worth. And one of the implications of this is that the prescribed boundaries of selfhood have become limited to what is seen as the ideal of 'the self-contained and self-controlled individual' (Crawford 1994: 1359). Individuals whose conduct is deemed contrary to the pursuit of a 'risk-free' existence are likely to be seen, and to see themselves, as lacking self-control, and as therefore not fulfilling their duties as fully autonomous, responsible citizens.

Greco points to the increasing trend for self-care to become a relevant variable in the economic rationale of private enterprises (Greco 1993: 369). In several countries, including Canada, the United States and Australia, firms are taking it upon themselves to define and manage health according to abstract calculations of risk. For example, stress prevention schemes which involve the establishment of personal risk profiles, on the basis of which individuals choose individually tailored programmes aimed at reducing personal risk, are becoming common. These schemes are seen to have the potential to offer financial savings for individual enterprises and the economy as a whole. For example, in early 1993, after the release of health expenditure figures showed an increase in health expenditure during the previous year, the Liberal government in New South Wales, Australia, sought a review of insurance companies' benefit tables to encourage more people to undertake preventive health measures such as visits to a gym or a nutritionist (Bita 1993: 2).

The privatisation of risk management has consequences for the kinds of relations one has with one's own self, with others, and with experts in particular. One is, first of all, called upon to be accountable to oneself; to continuously demonstrate to oneself one's competency to take care of the self and others. One may demonstrate one's accountability to one's self in a very public way through one's involvement in self-help groups or in processes for developing self-esteem. The health goals and targets proposal, mentioned above, refers to a number of specific proposals to improve self-esteem and skills in problem-solving, and to create opportunities to participate in self-help groups. For example, one of the goals is:

> to increase the proportion [of older people 60 years or more] who express confidence in their ability to manage stress associated with life events common to this stage of life (e.g. loss of a partner, relocation from a house to supported accommodation).

Another is:

> to increase the proportion [of the total population] who can provide simple support to one another at times of intense distress and crisis by: for example, allowing the person to express distress; being there for the person at time of need and caring compassionately for them.
> (Commonwealth of Australia 1993: 160–1)

That the development of individual 'life skills' is seen to mesh with the broader goal of promoting the social good is apparent in this quote:

> there is evidence that individuals whose self-esteem is high, who are able to communicate well with others, who are integrated into community networks of their choosing, and who have problem-solving and conflict resolution skills, generally have greater capacity to take action to promote and protect personal health, and to participate in collective problem solving and action to improve the health of communities.
> (Commonwealth of Australia 1993: 158)

Demonstration to oneself and others of one's ability to care for oneself is evident in such risk-minimisation practices as meditation, moderation, abstention, attention to diet and exercise. Many of these practices are premised on the idea of the body as a commodity that can be reshaped according to fashion, and the consumer's 'will power' and ability to purchase the range of expertise and tools now available in the 'body industry' (Koval 1986). The kind of detailed work on the self that this requires can be seen in the case of the pursuit of 'fitness'. Fitness is widely promoted as an opportunity to avert several of the risks to selfhood present in modern society; a way to protect oneself from characteristic ills of modern culture such as drug abuse, depression, eating disorders and cardiovascular disease (Glassner 1989: 180–91). And, among other things, this requires the individual to constantly monitor body 'inputs' (e.g. attention to diet, sleep and consumption of such 'unhealthy' products as tobacco, alcohol, fast foods) and 'outputs' (time-management, heart rate, muscle size, body shape and weight). In a culture in which physical appearance is seen as an important means of claiming status, health promotion feeds into, and reinforces, the 'cult of the body' whereby the striving after a 'risk-free' existence may mean, among other things, a great expenditure of time and energy on individualised fitness programmes, exercise equipment for home use, strict diet regimes, cosmetic surgery and so on (Finkelstein 1991: 2–4).

Some forms of body management, such as excessive exercise and some diets, far from protecting the self from 'risk', may in themselves constitute something of a hazard. This is particularly so in those cases where the pursuit of the ideal 'risk-free' state reaches obsessive proportions and leads to such forms of compulsive behaviour as 'exercise addiction' or anorexia. In the case of exercise addiction, although restricted to a relatively small proportion of all exercisers, the condition has affected so many individuals in absolute terms that a number of hospitals and health foundations have been obliged to establish units aimed at helping compulsive exercisers to exercise less (Dutton 1995: 275). Some forms of work on the self involve personal disclosures that are not only painful in themselves, but also make one vulnerable to public condemnation and ridicule, again with possibly lasting effects. The self-esteem movement, spearheaded by Gloria Steinem, involves getting people to publicly confess personal struggles with their lack of self-esteem, and programme goals include 'getting clients to write and tell their personal narratives with an eye to the public good' (Cruikshank 1993: 329). Self-esteem is linked to social goals such as amelioration of poverty, crime and gender inequality. And those who fail to make this link are likely to be charged with 'anti-social behaviour' and as 'lacking self-esteem' (Cruikshank 1993: 330). As Cruikshank points out, self-esteem advocates seem not to recognise the extent to which personal life is a product of power relations (1993: 341).

EXPERTISE AND THE ILLUSION OF ULTIMATE SECURITY

One of the ironies of risk discourse is that while it carries the promise of ultimate security, the 'free market' of expertise generates its own uncertainties. Different groups have different interests in promoting their own risk narratives. In the area of risk assessment there is much disagreement between experts: about what constitutes a risk, levels of risk, how to respond and so on. For example, there has been a long-standing debate among experts about whether or not electro-magnetic radiation from electric transmission lines poses a threat to those living in the vicinity and, if it does, what level of exposure is hazardous. Electricity authorities and groups of residents who live in proximity to transmission lines are bound to promote different risk narratives. There may be consensus about the existence of risk, but divided opinion on the level and/or source of risk. This is evident in respect to the issue of lead in the environment: experts seem to agree there is a health risk, but disagree about the level of risk and about whether the primary environmental source of lead in the blood is paint or petrol. There is also much conflicting advice about preventive measures: levels of required fitness, whether abstention or moderation is called for, or individual or structural change, and so on. Dietary advice is but one area replete with conflicting claims: for example, the merits of vegetarianism and of high fibre diets, 'safe' levels of cholesterol and alcohol intake, the dangers of eating snacks and fast foods, and the value of fasting. Although one of the underlying assumptions of health promotion is that science can discover objective, ultimate truths about risk and provide a basis for making ethical decisions about personal conduct, it is evident that scientists themselves cannot agree on the 'facts' about risk.

Scientists frequently disagree among themselves about the meaning and significance of statistical correlations upon which the calculation of factors of risk are based. Again, this is apparent in the lead debate, where there have been disagreements over the statistical relationship between lead in the blood and IQ levels in children, which is a measure commonly used to assess health impacts of lead. One scientist has even suggested that the relationship between lead in the blood and IQ is that 'children with a lower IQ are slower to grow out of the habit of putting things in their mouth' (Legge 1993: 23). Disagreement among experts means that there are rarely coherent sets of norms to which one may defer in caring for oneself. The ever-changing definitions of risk, which occur even as the changes in lifestyle that were called for are adopted, draw attention to the highly tentative nature of risk prediction and prevention. As Giddens points out, smoking was once advocated by some sectors of the medical profession as a relaxant, while red meat, butter and cream were strongly advocated as 'healthy' products (Giddens 1991: 121). Yet, according to the dictates of contemporary health promotion, all these products are factors of risk and should therefore be limited or avoided. There has been some recent scientific evidence challenging the benefits of vigorous exercise in promoting health. Claims that moderate regular exercise may be a more beneficial preventive strategy than short-term intense workouts serve to cast some doubt on earlier scientific claims about ideal levels of aerobic fitness and health. Similarly, concern expressed about the adverse health affects of water fluoridation and of aluminium-treated water, common in Australia and New Zealand respectively, has opened some space for the questioning of scientific assumptions underlying these public health measures for preventing dental disease (Kawachi and Pearce 1991; McMichael and Slade 1991). Conflicting and changing advice about sources and levels of risk means that the individual consumer of expert advice can never know for certain whether any particular set of advice is more likely to guarantee security than any another.

CONCLUSION

This chapter has sought to explore the utility of the concepts of risk and governance, as developed by Foucauldian scholars, in the analysis of health promotion strategies of the new public health. I began the argument by pointing out that recent thinking in the sociology of risk has tended to be dominated by the ideas of Anthony Giddens and Ulrich Beck, who share a similar perspective on risk and uncertainty in late modern society. I pointed to some problems and limitations with this work, which are related to these writers' adherence to conventional, modernist notions of self, science and society. Within the Giddens–Beck schema, the self is posited as an autonomous, 'reflexive' entity, and there is little acknowledgement of the role of expertise in regulating subjectivity. The work of Robert Castel and other governmentality theorists, focusing as it does on the political rationalities of the contemporary period, recognises a more complexly structured and intensely governed self.

As Turner, and Bunton and Petersen, note above (in the 'Foreword' and 'Introduction', respectively), Foucault's concept of governmentality can be conceived as a contact point between technologies of the self

(self-subjection) and technologies of domination (societal regulation). It allows one to recognise the agency of subjects, without recourse to the notion of a fully autonomous self or to voluntaristic explanations of behaviour. In the analysis of risk, it shifts the focus from uncertainties and dilemmas associated with individual 'life-planning' and 'lifestyle choice' (evident in the accounts of Giddens and Beck) to an analysis of 'practices of the self' and modes of self-subjection. The new public health can be seen to comprise a multiplicity of suggested practices, which provide potential points of reference for individuals in constituting themselves as subjects. In a 'neo-liberal' context, many of the practices of the new public health would seem to be closely aligned to the development described by Gordon as the 'managerialization of personal identity and personal relations' (1991: 44). This entails, among other things, the widespread tendency to establish links between personal goals and 'the public good', evident in the aforementioned 'self-esteem movement', and the tendency for individuals to be evaluated according to their abilities to effectively regulate themselves and others in line with prescribed norms of conduct for 'healthy living'. As I argued in this chapter, 'risk' would seem to play a crucial role in 'neo-liberal' societies: in distancing experts from direct intervention into personal lives, while employing the agency of subjects in their own self-regulation ('risk management'). It would be wrong, however, to assume (as modernist theorists of power tend to do) that domination of subjects is complete and coercive, and always involves techniques of rational control. The governmentality concept allows one to acknowledge the complexities, subtleties and micro-negotiations of relations of power, and involves recognition that any project of governance is always incomplete and partial in respect to the objects and practices it governs (Malpas and Wickham 1995). (Osborne's comments about the indeterminacy of health policy are relevant in this respect; see chapter 9.)

Critics of the new public health have so far emphasised the individualism, behaviourism, consumerism, and 'victim-blaming' associated with the lifestyle emphasis of health promotion (e.g. Bunton *et al.* 1995; Lupton 1995). As yet, there has been relatively little exploration of the processes of self-subjection associated with the multiple imperatives of public health. With the recent and considerable broadening of the mandate of public health to include the strategies of 'community participation', 'green politics', 'sustainable development', 'intersectoral collaboration' and 'healthy public policy', individuals are being called upon to play an increasingly active role in creating a 'healthy', 'sustainable' environment. The emergence of the new public health would seem to signal a new politics of citizenship, with a greater emphasis on 'duties implied by rights' (Roche 1992). Being a 'healthy', 'responsible', citizen entails new kinds of detailed work on the self and new interpersonal demands and responsibilities. The strategy of 'community participation', universally applauded by new public health commentators as the means of 'empowering' citizens, establishes its own disciplines of the self (e.g. the requirement that one engage with formal political structures and with various experts, and the ability to demonstrate commitment to shared goals and to manage interpersonal conflict), and may serve as a strategy of exclusion (Petersen 1996; Petersen and Lupton 1996). As Lupton points out in her study of patient–doctor interactions above (chapter 5), engagements with experts also involve complex negotiations of power at the interpersonal level – often entailing emotional or 'unconscious' (i.e. non-rational) elements. These complexities and micro-dynamics of relations of power have barely begun to be explored in the critical literature on the new public health, but can begin to be examined within the governmentality framework.

This chapter has discussed some implications of recent developments in the new public health, focusing in particular on the so-called health goals and targets strategy of health promotion and on a number of emergent practices of 'self-help' and 'care of the self'. However, there is a need for a more thoroughgoing enquiry into the other aspects of the new public health, such as those mentioned above. The work of Castel and other Foucauldian scholars who have developed the notions of risk and governance, I believe, can be used to good effect by those seeking to appraise the impact of the strategies of the new public health on everyday life.

NOTE

An earlier version of this chapter first appeared in *The Australian and New Zealand Journal of Sociology*, 32, 1 (1996): 44–57.

REFERENCES

Ashton, J. (ed.) (1992) *Healthy Cities*, Buckingham: Open University Press.
Ashton, J. and Seymour, H. (1988) *The New Public Health: The Liverpool Experience*, Milton Keynes: Open University Press.
Beck, U. (1992) *Risk Society: Towards a New Modernity*, London: Sage.
Beck, U. (1995) *Ecological Politics in an Age of Risk*, Cambridge: Polity Press.

Beck, U., Giddens, A. and Lash, S. (1994) *Reflexive Modernization: Politics, Tradition and Aesthetics in the Modern Social Order*, Cambridge: Polity Press.

Bita, N. (1993) 'Bid for fitness bonus under private cover', *The Australian*, 30 April: 2.

Bunton, R. (1992) 'More than a woolly jumper: health promotion as social regulation', *Critical Public Health*, 3, 2: 4–11.

Bunton, R., Nettleton, S. and Burrows, R. (1995) *The Sociology of Health Promotion: Critical Analyses of Consumption, Lifestyle and Risk*, London: Routledge.

Burchell, G. (1993) 'Liberal government and techniques of the self', *Economy and Society*, 22, 3: 267–82.

Castel, R. (1991) 'From dangerousness to risk', in G. Burchell, C. Gordon and P. Miller (eds), *The Foucault Effect: Studies in Governmentality*, Hemel Hempstead: Harvester Wheatsheaf.

Commonwealth of Australia (1993) *Goals and Targets for Australia's Health in the Year 2000 and Beyond*, Report prepared for the Commonwealth Department of Health, Housing and Community Services by D. Nutbeam, M. Wise, A. Bauman, E. Harris and S. Leeder, Department of Public Health, University of Sydney, Canberra: AGPS.

Commonwealth of Australia (1994) *Better Health Outcomes for Australians: National Goals, Targets and Strategies for Better Health Outcomes into the Next Century*, Canberra: AGPS.

Crawford, R. (1994) 'The boundaries of the self and the unhealthy other: reflections on health, culture and AIDS', *Social Science and Medicine*, 38, 10: 1347–65.

Cruikshank, B. (1993) 'Revolutions within: self-government and self-esteem', *Economy and Society*, 22, 3: 327–44.

Davies, J.K. and Kelly, M. (1993) *Healthy Cities: Research and Practice*, London: Routledge.

Douglas, M. (1990) 'Risk as a forensic resource', *Daedalus*, 119, 4: 1–16.

Douglas, M. (1992) *Risk and Blame: Essays in Cultural Theory*, London: Routledge.

Douglas, M. and Wildavsky, A. (1982) *Risk and Culture*, Oxford: Basil Blackwell.

Dutton, K.R. (1995) *The Perfectible Body: The Western Ideal of Physical Development*, London: Cassell.

Ewald, F. (1991) 'Insurance and risk', in G. Burchell, C. Gordon and P. Miller (eds) *The Foucault Effect: Studies in Governmentality*, London: Harvester Wheatsheaf.

Finkelstein, J. (1991) *The Fashioned Self*, Cambridge: Polity Press.

Foucault, M. (1991) 'Governmentality', in G. Burchell, C. Gordon and P. Miller (eds) *The Foucault Effect: Studies in Governmentality*, London: Harvester Wheatsheaf.

Freeman, R. (1991) 'The idea of prevention: a critical review', in S. Scott, G. Williams, S. Platt and H. Thomas (eds) *Private Risks and Public Dangers*, Aldershot: Avebury.

Fujimura, J.H. and Chou, D.Y. (1994) 'Dissent in science: styles of scientific practice and the controversy over the cause of AIDS', *Social Science and Medicine*, 38, 8: 1017–35.

206 Alan Petersen

Giddens, A. (1991) *Modernity and Self-Identity: Self and Society in the Late Modern Age*, Stanford: Stanford University Press.

Glassner, B. (1989) 'Fitness and the postmodern self', *Journal of Health and Social Behaviour*, 30, 2: 180–91.

Gordon, C. (1991) 'Governmental rationality: an introduction', in G. Burchell, C. Gordon and P. Miller (eds) *The Foucault Effect: Studies in Governmentality*, Hemel Hempstead: Harvester Wheatsheaf.

Greco, M. (1993) 'Psychosomatic subjects and the "duty to be well": personal agency within medical rationality', *Economy and Society*, 22, 3: 357–72.

Kawachi, I. and Pearce, N. (1991) 'Aluminium in the drinking water – is it safe?', *Australian Journal of Public Health*, 15, 2: 84–7.

Koval, R. (1986) *Eating Your Heart Out: Food, Shape and the Body Industry*, Ringwood: Penguin.

Labonte, R. (1990) 'Empowerment: notes on professional and community, dimensions', *Canadian Review of Social Policy*, 26: 64–75.

Lash, S. (1994) 'Reflexivity and its doubles: structure, aesthetics, community', in U. Beck, A. Giddens and S. Lash *Reflexive Modernization: Politics, Tradition and Aesthetics in the Modern Social Order*, Cambridge: Polity Press.

Lash, S. and Urry, J. (1994) *Economies of Signs and Space*, London: Sage.

Legge, K. (1993) 'High octane handicap', *The Weekend Australian*, 24–5 July: 23.

Luhmann, N. (1993) *Risk: A Sociological Theory*, New York: Walter de Gruyter.

Lupton, D. (1995) *The Imperative of Health: Public Health and the Regulated Body*, London: Sage.

Malpas, J. and Wickham, G. (1995) 'Governance and failure: on the limits of sociology', *Australian & New Zealand Journal of Sociology*, 31, 3: 37–50.

McMichael, A.J. and Slade, G.D. (1991) 'An element of dental health? Fluoride and dental disease in contemporary Australia', *Australian Journal of Public Health*, 15, 2: 80–3.

Petersen, A.R. (1996) 'The "healthy" city, expertise, and the regulation of space', *Health and Place: An International Journal*, 2, 3: 157–65.

Petersen, A.R. and Lupton, D. (1996) *The New Public Health: Health and Self in the Age of Risk*, Sydney: Allen and Unwin, and London: Sage.

Roche, M. (1992) *Rethinking Citizenship: Welfare, Ideology and Change in Modern Society*, Cambridge: Polity Press.

Rose, N. (1993) 'Government, authority and expertise in advanced liberalism', *Economy and Society*, 22, 3: 283–99.

Rose, N. and Miller, P. (1992) 'Political power beyond the state: problematics of government', *British Journal of Sociology*, 43, 2: 173–205.

Scott, S. and Williams, G. (1991) 'Introduction', in S. Scott, G. Williams, S. Platt and H. Thomas (eds) *Private Risks and Public Dangers*, Aldershot: Avebury.

Wallerstein, N. (1993) 'Empowerment and health: the theory and practice of community change', *Community Development Journal*, 28, 3: 218–27.

Yeo, M. (1993) 'Toward an ethic of empowerment for health promotion', *Health Promotion International*, 8, 3: 225–35.

Chapter 11

Governing the risky self
How to become healthy, wealthy and wise

Sarah Nettleton

The *Sunday Times* in association with PPP Healthcare and the publishers Dorling Kindersley published, in early 1996, a series of six pamphlets entitled *Change Your Life: A Six-part Guide to Health and Diet*. John Witherow, the editor of the *Sunday Times*, prefaced the first edition:

> It is time to take action. To change your life. The new year is the perfect moment to make the most important resolution of your life – to be healthier in mind and body. This week *The Sunday Times* launches an essential six-part guide to living better and living longer. Over the next six weeks, our experts will advise you on all aspects of healthy eating and living. We do not offer food fads or instant solutions, but simple, sensible ways to take control of your life. We will not preach about the improbable and the impossible, but talk about the probable and the possible. It's you who can make a difference.
>
> Learn how to adopt a realistic eating plan; find out which 'power foods' can help prevent some illnesses; work out how to get the most from a fitness regime, whether you are a signed-up jogger or a self-declared exercise phobe; understand the techniques that can help you beat stress before it becomes a problem. . . .
>
> It is time to change your life for the better and the good. *The Sunday Times* has joined forces with PPP Healthcare and Dorling Kindersley, the leading publisher of health books, to bring you this indispensable six-part series – specially designed so that you can take control of your most valuable resource. Your health.
>
> (Witherow 1996: 1)

This publication is, in a number of ways, emblematic of contemporary approaches to health and health care. First, it is produced by private commercial companies. PPP Healthcare obviously have an interest in ensuring that people invest in their own health, Dorling Kindersley are likely to want to increase their sales of the ever-growing number of books on maintaining health, and the *Sunday Times* presumably feel that health is a newsworthy issue with which people are keen to engage. Second, Witherow points out that the intention is not to 'preach'; rather information will be provided (or promoted?) about the 'probable and the possible' so that readers can make their own choices and tailor the information to their own personal health needs. Third, the emphasis is on lifestyle factors which are associated with good health rather than medical and technical interventions. Fourth, the information will be provided by 'experts', which implies that it will be based on objective and scientific knowledge. Fifth, there is the suggestion that it is possible for 'you', that is the individual, to be in control over his or her destiny; it is the individual who is best able to effect change to make his or her life 'better'.

Today health and health care is identified with more than hospitals and medical bureaucracies; health matters are to be found in a whole array of agencies, institutions and settings. Health maintenance involves the consumption of a range of goods and services which are increasingly marketed for their health-giving properties, such as food, exercise machines and fitness clubs. Health is something which lies within the control of the individual. All active citizens have a right and a duty to maintain, contribute to and ensure (or should that be insure?) their health status. Health, like other aspects of welfare, is something which is not maintained by state-provided bureaucracies. For example, in recent years individuals have been encouraged to purchase their own private pensions and tailor them to their personal needs and circumstances. Similarly, in the UK when buying a house, the changes in legislation to social security payments on the mortgage payments mean that individuals are encouraged to take out personal protection plans in case of adversity. The point is that contemporary forms of welfare are increasingly requiring that individuals take personal responsibility for their own future and purchase goods and services which are designed to meet their personal requirements. A range of risks are presented by the 'experts' and it is up to individuals to calculate the likely consequences of certain actions for themselves.

The de-collectivisation of welfare, the rise of personal responsibility for future security and health, and the expansion of markets and consumption into areas which, since the Second World War, had been provided by state monopolies can be accounted for in a number of ways. First, and somewhat crudely, there is a political economy perspective which would draw attention to the changing nature of contemporary capitalism, which, with the move from a Fordist to post-Fordist era, requires not only the expansion of markets for a wider range of services but also the need for more distinctive and focused marketing. Healthy profits can indeed be made from health. Second, there is an ideological approach which would privilege the importance of the beliefs, values and philosophy of the New Right and point to its incessant determination to dismantle those forms of welfare which have been established over the past five decades. These explanations, which are well known and have been well documented, are instructive as they provide insights into the economic and political processes which have brought about such developments. This chapter, however, wants to tell a different story.

Drawing on the work of Foucault, a number of authors (Hewitt 1991; Squires 1990) have provided alternative accounts of such events and are particularly valuable in terms of understanding many of the key characteristics of contemporary approaches and preoccupations within current discourses on health. These characteristics (evident in our *Sunday Times* pamphlet) are: the active individual or 'the self'; the salience of 'expertise'; and the unshakeable belief that our quality of life can be 'better'. It has been argued further that contemporary forms of liberal democratic government presuppose a certain conceptualisation of 'self': a self that is autonomous, subjective and active (Rose 1990, 1992). A corollary to this is that the activities and practices of government contribute to the constitution of such subjects and subjectivity. This 'Foucauldian' account is different to the two others mentioned above in that it argues that the techniques and practices of experts in the human sciences (psychology, sociology, medicine, etc.) are critical to the possibility of contemporary forms of health and welfare. It further suggests that such developments are not merely a function of dominant ideological forms but rather the 'mentalities of government' (Rose 1992) which transcend them. It also acknowledges the salience of self-government in modern society. This form of analysis is useful in that it reveals the significance of the knowledge, activities and tasks of health professionals or psychologists to the formation of prevailing notions of the self, which in turn is pivotal to the nature of modern forms of welfare.

Nikolas Rose (1990, 1992) has most usefully articulated the conceptualisation of 'the self', which in turn is, he argues, inseparable from modern forms of 'government'. Rose and others (Greco 1993;

Ogden 1995) have also pointed to the importance of the 'psychological sciences' in establishing the predominant notion of the subjective self. This notion of the active self is especially critical in the light of the explosion within the epidemiological and medical literature of risk factors associated with health over which the individual can have some control. Finally, by drawing on these studies which have been informed by Foucault's writings, this chapter hopes to demonstrate not only that such approaches provide valuable accounts of the emergence of current forms of health and health care, but also that Foucauldian analyses are not, as some authors have suggested, invariably gloomy, nor do they imply that humans are trapped in a web of surveillance and social control which encroaches ever further into their physical, psychological and social lives.

THE GOVERNMENT OF SUBJECTS

When articulating his ideas on government Foucault draws a distinction between sovereign rule – the submission of people to the rule of law – and 'the art of government', which involves the exercise of power which does not concern so much the protection of territory, but rather the protection of individuals and the population to ensure their security in terms of their wealth, resources, health, happiness and so on. Foucault (1979: 20) defines government thus:

> the ensemble formed by the institutions, procedures, analyses and reflections, the calculations and tactics that allow the exercise of this very specific albeit complex form of power, which has as its target population, as its principal form of knowledge political economy and its essential technical means apparatuses of security.

Political thought or the mentality of government since the eighteenth century has been primarily concerned with the population (its object) and the economic and social health and well-being of the individuals of which it is comprised (its subjects). Foucault points out that the activities of government and the state are predominantly those of collecting, collating and calculating data on the characteristics of the population (births, deaths, rates of disease, levels and types of employment, etc.). He also emphasises that these institutional activities are complemented by those of individuals who engage in practices of the self or 'self-government'. Individuals shape their own lives as well as react to the influence and actions of others:

the subject constitutes himself [sic] in an active fashion, by the practices of self, these practices are nevertheless not something that the individual invents by himself. They are patterns that he finds in his culture and which are proposed, suggested and imposed on him by his culture, his society and his social group.

(Foucault 1988: 11)

The art of government therefore requires and develops a knowledge of its population and the families and individuals of which it is comprised. It gathers and calculates data to ensure that the government is effective and capable in achieving the ends of establishing a healthy, happy, and productive population. Foucault identifies the salience of what he refers to as 'pastoral power' to this form of governance. Pastoral power is critical to this conceptualisation of governance, not least because of its techniques of individualisation. Foucault (1982: 783) notes that the concept of pastorship within the context of early Christianity had four characteristics: it assures individual salvation; it does not just command sacrifice (like royal power) but must also be prepared to make sacrifices for subjects; it looks after each and every individual for his or her whole life; and it exercises the need to know people's minds, souls, secrets and details of their actions. Although the institutionalisation of Christianity diminished during the eighteenth century, the state still functioned as 'a modern matrix of pastoral power'. Pastoral power no longer implies, of course, that individuals be led to salvation, but rather that they be assured of other worldly goods such as health, well-being and security. In tandem with this change, the officials of pastoral power, who were previously members of religious institutions, 'spread into a whole social body' and 'found support in a multitude of institutions' such as 'those of the family, medicine, psychiatry, education and employers' (Foucault 1982).

In sum, here government refers to all those ways in which the economic, social and personal aspects of our lives are administered: the systems of data collection and the policies and programmes which, based upon this data, are designed to ensure the well-being of the object of government – the population – and its subjects – individuals; governance which deploys a technique of power which Foucault calls pastoral power, an individualising form of power which requires a detailed knowledge of the mental and physical attributes of its subjects.

This form of power cannot be exercised without knowing the inside of people's minds, without exploring their souls, without making them reveal their innermost secrets. It implies a knowledge of the conscience and an ability to direct it.

(Foucault 1982: 783)

This in turn requires that individuals learn how to know themselves. Rose (1990) has provided a detailed analysis of the 'experts' of the human 'soul' who have arisen during the twentieth century within the contexts of the world wars, work and the family. These 'experts' assist in the process of understanding the self. Government has increasingly come to rely on these 'technologies of the self' to shape and enhance the capacities of individuals. The subjects of government within this context are autonomous, independent and self-reliant. As Rose (1992) argues in the paper 'Governing the enterprising self', this type of self accords with the prevailing political values of our time. As Rose explains, in advanced liberal democracies subjects are not required to fulfil duties and obligations but are endowed with rights and freedoms. He writes:

the presupposition of the autonomous, choosing, free self as the value, ideal and objective underpinning and legitimating political activity imbues the political mentalities of the modern West.

(1992: 142)

Government does not just subject its subjects to policies and programmes but requires that they participate. Individuals are recruited to take care of themselves, but the techniques that are deployed by the 'experts' of human conduct must in turn invariably shape how individuals come to think about them*selves*.

In this sense, through the mechanisms of government, the self is fundamentally related to power. Rose (1992: 143–5) suggests that these relations can be explored along three interlinked dimensions: political, institutional and ethical. The 'political' dimension highlights the extent to which the capacities of subjects or citizens form both a target and a resource for political authorities (in ways described above). Forms of political rule are inextricably interlinked with conceptions of those who are to be ruled (Rose 1992: 144). The 'institutional' dimension refers to those sites or organisations where practices are undertaken which work upon the individuals or the selves who are associated with them. (This is of course most readily evident in Foucault's 1977 study of prisons.) The 'ethical' dimension refers to the 'means by which individuals come to construe, decipher and act upon themselves in relation to the true and the false, the permitted and the forbidden, the desirable and the undesirable' (Rose 1992: 144). In other words, governance functions at the levels of political rhetoric, institutional practice and individual conscience. The values which influence how we are governed overlap with those which shape how we govern ourselves; they are those which privilege the independent self. Such a self, according to Rose, has been forged by the 'experts' of the mind; the range of 'professionals' who are involved with psychotherapeutics.

> The codes and vocabularies of psychotherapeutics thus can bring into alignment the techniques for the regulation of subjectivity and the technologies of government elaborated within contemporary political rationales. It promises to make it possible for us all to make a project of our biography, create a style for our lives, shape our everyday existence in terms of an ethic of autonomy.
>
> (Rose 1990: 254)

Returning to the example of health, it is conceived within political rhetoric and practices that it is possible to influence one's own trajectory and to make one's body and lifestyle a project. For example, in the introduction to the *Health of the Nation* consultation document, William Waldegrave (Department of Health 1991: v) notes that:

> You cannot in the end coerce people into good health. That is why we need mutual agreement on priorities and on how best to work together to improve health. . . . Implementation depends, in the current jargon, on shared 'ownership'.

As we have thus far argued, this turns on certain presuppositions of the notion of self as autonomous, capable and free thinking which have been evident in a range of settings, such as the workplace, where psychotherapeutics got a grip. Such a notion of the self is, however, especially poignant in relation to health, as there has been a proliferation in the range of 'health risks' over which an individual can now take action to 'insure' against disease or illness.

HEALTH, RISK AND THE AUTONOMOUS SELF

A number of authors (Arney and Bergen 1984; Nettleton 1989; Greco 1993; Ogden 1995) have demonstrated how, within the discourse of health and health care, psychological theories and practices have contributed to the reconfiguration of the individual, or subject, from being a relatively 'docile', passive recipient of advice and health care to one who possesses the capacity for self-control, responsibility, rationality and enterprise. Greco (1993) demonstrates how those writing on the subject of 'psychosomatics' drew attention to those internal (psychological and cognitive) psycho-social factors which affect health. Such factors complement 'external' factors such as age, social class, sex, marital status and so on. The monitoring of the individuals therefore cannot be limited to 'an objective environment or . . . a body-object' (Greco 1993: 361) but must also seek out the subjective truth of a body capable of consciousness. Accordingly risk is determined not only by one's personal circumstances but also one's personal *capacities*.

> Each individual thus acquires a personal preventive capacity *vis-à-vis* the event of his or her illness, a preventive capacity structured around the possibility of self-transformation and, before that, of self knowledge. If the regulation of life-style, the modification of risky behaviour and the transformation of unhealthy attitudes prove impossible through sheer strength of will, this constitutes, at least in part, a *failure of the self to take care of itself* – a form of irrationality, or simply a lack of *skilfulness*. . . . The mastery of the self is thus a prerequisite for health; the lack of self-mastery, accordingly, is a 'disease' prior to the actual physical complaint, whose symptoms are detectable as behaviourial, psychological and cognitive patterns.
>
> (Greco 1993: 361)

Ogden's (1995) analysis of the impact of psychological theory reaches a similar conclusion. It is not environmental factors, or bacteria or viruses *per se* that cause illness; the critical factor resides in individuals, more particularly their self control. '[C]ontemporary health risks . . . as indicated by the contemporary psychological literature are to be found within the self' (1995: 413). In fact, she points out, 'in the twentieth century the individual has become at risk from his or herself'. Echoing the work of Rose, both these authors argue that it is transformations in psychological thought and practice that has transformed notions of the self and identity. Such notions of the self-reliant and enterprising self are of course reflected in, and form a useful adjunct to, the ideology of the New Right, but its conditions of possibility are to be located more in the activities of the 'experts' of the human condition.

Just as the knowledge and activities of the 'human sciences' (psychology, therapeutics, medicine) have contributed to the transformation and the formation of an autonomous and independent self who is endowed with the capacities of choice and free will, they have also contributed to the formation and linkage to health and welfare of another notion, namely *risk*. As we discussed above, contemporary forms of welfare encourage individuals to insure their own futures, their security. The state cannot be relied upon to care for all our welfare needs, but individuals must draw upon the knowledge produced by the 'experts' to assess their futures and take control of their biography. Commenting on the work of Ewald (1991), Donzelot (1991) and Castel (1991), Greco (1993: 360) notes how: 'A conversion process in mental attitudes is taking place in line with what has recently been described as a philosophy of risk . . . in relation to the domains of insurance, work and mental medicine respectively.' Such a philosophy is also apparent in relation to physical medicine.

An analysis of medical journals in Britain, the USA and Scandinavia found that the increase in the use of the term 'risk' has reached 'epidemic' proportions (Skolbekken 1995). The study looked at journals published between 1967 and 1991; for the first five years the number of 'risk articles' published was around 1,000 and for the last five years there were over 80,000. Skolbekken suggests that health promotion provides 'the ideological frame needed to explain the present emphasis on factors regarded as risks to our health. . . . Through the ideological frame of health promotion we get a glimpse of some of the functions served by the risk epidemic' (1995: 296). These functions are identified as, first, to predict disease and death, in other words to gain control over disease which in turn confirms our faith in medical science. Second, the findings of this type of research may help to save money as people are less likely to require acute and therefore expensive services. Third, it contributes to 'medicalisation'. Risk factors which are hypothesised to be linked to disease come to be treated as 'diseases to be cured'.

The selection and confirmation of such risk factors is often subject to controversy and the evidence about causal links is often not unequivocal, but the point to be made here is that the emphasis on risk factors which are within the control of the individual contributes to the confirmation of the active citizen, the self who can be, and indeed *ought* to be, in control of his or her self. It may impact upon one's social identity in that one is not well, not ill but 'at risk' (Davison *et al.* 1994: 355). The recourse to epidemiology by those involved in the promotion of health is invaluable as it provides a veneer of scientific legitimacy, objectivity and expertise (Lupton 1995: 67).

Rose (1992: 148) argues that such 'expertise' is important to the exercise of power (i.e. conduct of conduct) in at least three respects. First, by locating the authority of claims in 'scientificity' this serves to distance systems of self-regulation from formal forms of political power. Second, 'expertise' can be mobilised within political argument wherein it can play a particular role in the development of programmes of government. Third, expertise has a salience for the 'self-regulating capacities of subjects' in that it ties their subjectivity to 'truth' and in this respect it has a potent ethical dimension. In turn, a recourse to expertise can also mean that subjects may form new relationships with 'experts' (we return to this point on p. 219). Individuals are not, then, simply told how to behave; they are also provided with expert knowledge upon which they must draw to suit their own particular health needs. This is done voluntarily and the marketisation of health products enables individuals (or at least those with resources) to select the ideal health package. Health promoters seek to equip those who do not have the resources with the skills to enable them to negotiate more 'healthy' lifestyles and discriminate between 'healthy' and 'unhealthy' activities. Thus there is a range of expert advisers who can provide us with an array of likely outcomes if we take certain actions.

Although the relative merits of routine screening programmes of healthy individuals have been questioned, in an era of uncertainty the 'security' of a health 'check up' may appear attractive to health planners, consumers and the private health care industry. Indeed, for some it must – in 1994 private health screens generated £31 million within the private health care sector (Illman 1996). But most people do not simply passively accept the pronouncements of medical 'experts' who may be equipped with varying forms of technological equipment; these are simply resources which individuals or 'consumers' are able to draw upon, or reject, when reflecting upon their lifestyles. Government requires the 'risky selves' to be wise about their investments for their future health and for their future wealth. For example, like the 'independent financial adviser', the expert health adviser sets out on his or her stall a number of possibilities from which we can select the most suitable and profitable 'investment'. Governments, policy-makers and other institutions and agencies can provide the 'facts' but ultimately it is individuals who decide, select and act upon them.

Government of population and self-governance does not, then, rely on certainties and unequivocal decisions. There is a persistent repicrocity between aggregate and individual actions, the consequences of which are not immediate and predictable, nor are they always clear cut. They take place in a wider social and economic context which remains untamed and uncertain. Such uncertainties might explain, in part, the current vogue for the identification of clear cut and definitive outcomes and evidence to demonstrate the effectiveness of interventions which in turn have resource implications. The promotion of health, like the promotion of wealth, is a tricky area when dealing with populations. This conundrum is acknowledged by a health promotion specialist during an interview with the author (Author's data, 1995) when she explained:

> I'm trying to argue that health promotion is not so much intervention as an investment and it should be looked at almost in parallel to the money market, where you put something in and you don't see very much coming back for some considerable time, but you can see where you've put it and you can see things beginning to happen, but you're not going to actually get your return for some period of time, which is longer than a financial year.

POWER AND CHANGE

Discourses on health and health policy presuppose a self that is able to react to and challenge 'expert' knowledge. Power is only effective if the subjects of power are able to react in a range of ways. It does not suppose, as has often been suggested, that individuals are passive, 'docile' and shaped by an all-embracing and consistent machinery of power. Foucault makes this quite clear.

> When one defines the exercise of power as a mode of action upon the action of others, when one characterises these actions by the government of men by other men [sic] . . . one includes an important element: freedom. Power is exercised only over free subjects, and only in so far as they are free. By this we mean individual or collective subjects who are faced with a field of possibilities in which several ways of behaving, several reactions and diverse compartments, may be realised. Where the determining factors saturate the whole, there is no relationship of power; slavery is not a power relationship when man [sic] is in chains.
>
> (Foucault 1982: 790)

It is important to appreciate this quality of this conceptualisation of power; otherwise we would not be able to account for, one, any possibility of change and, two, the fact that individuals consistently are questioning and contesting power. For example, it is quite evident that knowledge and information about health and medicine are not simply formulated by medical experts (clinicians, scientists, etc.) and disseminated to a wider audience of health professionals and the public, who in turn accept them as a matter of course. Rather, the knowledge that is generated in these and other locations provides a valuable tool of government at the levels of political discourse, institutions and individuals. Here it may form a valuable dimension of the exercise of power. It may be critical to the function of power to 'a relationship which is at the same time reciprocal incitation and struggle, less of a face-to-face confrontation which paralyses both sides than a permanent provocation' (Foucault 1982: 790).

Government in this context is a dynamic process whereby the production and dissemination of information opens up new forms of knowledge and new styles of action. Given the current style of government is such that the autonomous, enterprising self is presumed and incited, the proliferation of activities to support such individuals is not surprising. Self-governance implies an ongoing project whereby we are continuously assessing information and expertise in relation to our selves. Giddens[1] refers to such activity as *reflexivity*, which he considers to be a key feature of modern society:

> The self today is for everyone a reflexive project – a more or less continuous interrogation of the past, present and future. It is a project carried on amid a profusion of reflexive resources: therapy and self-help manuals of all kinds, television programmes and magazine articles.
>
> (Giddens 1992: 30)

Giddens offers diet as a particularly pertinent example of this process of reflexivity. Significantly, in the *Sunday Times* pamphlets cited at the beginning of this chapter, most space was devoted to types of food and styles of eating which, it seems, are the cure for a myriad of ills and essential to the maintenance of health. As Giddens notes:

> The reflexivity of the body accelerates in a fundamental way with the invention of diet in its modern meaning. . . . Diet is linked to the introduction of a science of nutrition, and thus to administrative power in Foucault's sense; but it also places responsibility for the development and appearance of the body squarely in the hands of its possessor. What an individual eats, even among the more materially deprived, becomes a reflexively infused question of dietary selection. *Everyone* today in the developed countries, apart from the very poor, is on a diet. With the increased efficiency of global markets, not only is food abundant, but a diversity of foodstuffs is available for the consumer all year round. In these circumstances,

what one eats is a life-style choice, influenced by, and constructed through, vast numbers of cookbooks, popular medical tracts, nutritional guides and so forth.

(Giddens 1992: 31–2)

Commercialisation pervades the practices of self-governance and the governance of populations. Decisions made by individuals in the light of the multiplicity of sources of advice are made more complex in the light of the ever-expanding range of services and products or 'reflexive resources' (Giddens 1992: 32).

Amongst the general public there has been an increase in self-help groups around issues of health and medicine (Kelleher 1994); and amongst the media the number of magazines dealing with issues of health and fitness has soared. The marketisation of health is not, however, limited to the consumption of health products and health care that are not provided by the state. In the sphere of health policy there is a presumption that individuals are able to react to and contribute to policies. For example, in the UK health agencies are encouraged to, and have, put in place mechanisms to listen to 'local voices' (NHSME 1992) and ensure user involvement.

It seems that in general people tend to be 'ambivalent' about the value of modern medicine (Calnan and Williams 1996). When assessing their own lifestyles, individuals are discriminating in the way in which they assess information. For example, a study of lay views on coronary heart disease found that during discussions on such matters:

> Medical practitioners and researchers and health promotion authorities were also subjected to criticism [by patients/clients] based on the confusing messages evident in media accounts: 'even the most credible sources, like doctors, often come out with the most ridiculous things' (woman group 3).

(Lupton and Chapman 1995)

Lay perceptions of risk are not therefore simply moulded or influenced by those in 'authority' such as medical personnel, health promoters and policy-makers. As I mentioned above there may be new relationships between 'experts' and lay people as alliances are formed around disputes over particular cases and incidents.[2] Nor do people uniformly accept the pronouncements on health from other sources. For example, one morning whilst driving on a short journey I caught part of the *Midweek* discussion programme on BBC Radio 4 (20 March 1996). I gleaned from the discussion that one of the guests on the programme was a woman who experienced diabetes and epilepsy. During the conversation Libby Purves (the programme presenter) offered, with feeling, 'You read in all these magazines, it seems to be everywhere, that you must take control of your life, that you are responsible for your health, and you feel like saying "No I'm bloody not!" and throwing them across the room.' Amongst the group there seemed to be a degree of sympathy with this view, but the participants also appeared to agree that those people who were able to control their health and illness were to be admired, and that although you perhaps could not get better from a disease without medical help, there was much one could do to prevent its occurrence. Such tensions are also evident amongst those in positions of institutional 'authority' who would balk at the very suggestion that it is their place to 'tell' others how to behave to ensure their future health. Rather they would prefer to provide 'consumers', 'users' or whoever with information and a range of options so that they themselves can decide what is best for them. This requires that they draw on those specialist skills derived from the realms of psychotherapeutics, skills such as counselling. As a health promotion officer, during an interview with the author (1995), put it, 'I am from a counselling philosophy in that the person with whom they are working has the right to make up their own mind. I would stake my reputation on the fact that advice doesn't work.'

The enterprising, autonomous self is not just the creation of New Right ideology which privileges the individual over the social, and personal choice over collective consumption. It has in fact been forged out of the forms of governance which have drawn on 'expertise' – the knowledge and practices of the human sciences – especially psychology and sociology. Nevertheless, the conceptual fit is no doubt of value to those who want to pursue the marketisation of welfare for ideological purposes. Furthermore, the commercialisation of health and welfare invariably benefits from the formation of increasingly discriminating consumers of health care who also recognise that they can make informed investments for their future health. Clearly there is a reverberation between forms of governance located within state contexts and institutions and other non-state agencies and settings. Discourses and practices invariably transcend them. But the emergence of a person who acknowledges that he or she is able to contribute to his or her own health, wealth and well-being is part of wider shifts which are associated with the incessant change that is inevitable in, and necessary to, a society which is characterised by the play of what Foucault calls 'disciplinary power'.

NOTES

1 Although Giddens (1992) discusses Foucault's ideas, which he values not least for being so innovative, fundamentally he argues that Foucault's ideas are also 'deeply flawed'.
2 See, for example, Williams and Popay's (1994) analysis of the disputes surrounding the case of the spillage of aluminium sulphate solution in Camelford in the UK.

REFERENCES

Arney, W.R. and Bergen, B. (1984) *Medicine and the Management of Living: Taming the Last Great Beast*, London: University of Chicago Press.

Calnan, M. and Williams, S. (1996) 'Lay evaluation of scientific medicine and medical care', in S. Williams and M. Calnan (eds) *Modern Medicine: Lay Perspectives and Experiences*, London: University College London Press.

Castel, R. (1991) 'From dangerousness to risk', in G. Burchell, C. Gordon and P. Miller (eds) *The Foucault Effect: Studies in Governmentality*, London: Harvester Wheatsheaf.

Davison, C., Macintyre, S. and Davey Smith, G. (1994) 'The potential social impact of predictive genetic testing for susceptibility to common chronic diseases: a review and proposed research agenda', *Sociology of Health & Illness*, 16, 3: 340–71.

Department of Health (1991) *The Health of the Nation: A Consultation Document*, London: Department of Health.

Donzelot, J. (1991) 'The mobilisation of society', in G. Burchell, C. Gordon and P. Miller (eds) *The Foucault Effect: Studies in Governmentality*, London: Harvester Wheatsheaf.

Ewald, F. (1991) 'Insurance and risk', in G. Burchell, C. Gordon and P. Miller (eds) *The Foucault Effect: Studies in Governmentality*, London: Harvester Wheatsheaf.

Foucault, M. (1977) *Discipline and Punish. The Birth of the Prison*, London: Allen Lane.

Foucault, M. (1979) 'Governmentality', *Ideology and Consciousness*, 6: 5–22.

Foucault, M. (1982) 'The subject and power', *Critical Inquiry*, 8: 777–95.

Foucault, M. (1988) 'The ethic of care for the self as a practice of freedom', in J. Brenauer and D. Rasmussen (eds) *The Final Foucault*, Cambridge, Mass.: MIT Press.

Giddens, A. (1992) *The Transformation of Intimacy*, Cambridge: Polity Press.

Greco, M. (1993) 'Psychosomatic subjects and the "duty to be well": personal agency within medical rationality', *Economy and Society*, 22, 3: 357–72.

Hewitt, M. (1991) 'Bio-politics and social policy: Foucault's account of welfare', in M. Featherstone, M. Hepworth and B.S. Turner (eds) *The Body: Social Process and Cultural Theory*, London: Sage.

Illman, J. (1996) 'Fat fees and MOTs', *Guardian 2*, Tuesday 20 February: 11.

Kelleher, D. (1994) 'Self-help groups and their relationship to medicine', in J. Gabe, D. Kelleher and G. Williams (eds) *Challenging Medicine*, London: Routledge.

Lupton, D. (1995) *The Imperative of Health: Public Health and the Regulated Body*, London: Sage.

Lupton, D. and Chapman, S. (1995) 'A healthy lifestyle might be the death of you: discourses on diet, cholesterol control and heart disease in the press among lay people', *Sociology of Health & Illness*, 17, 4: 477–94.

Nettleton, S. (1989) 'Power and pain: the location of pain and fear in dentistry and the creation of the dental subject', *Social Science and Medicine*, 29, 10: 1183–90.

NHSME (National Health Service Management Executive) (1992) *Local Voices*, London: NHSME.

Ogden, J. (1995) 'Psychosocial theory and the creation of the risky self', *Social Science and Medicine*, 40, 3: 409–15.

Rose, N. (1990) *Governing the Soul: The Shaping of the Private Self*, London: Routledge.

Rose, N. (1992) 'Governing the enterprising self', in P. Heelas and P. Morris (eds) *The Values of the Enterprise Culture*, London: Routledge.

Squires, P. (1990) *Anti-Social Policy: Welfare, Ideology and the Disciplinary State*, London: Routledge.

Skolbekken, J. (1995) 'The risk epidemic in medical journals', *Social Science and Medicine*, 40, 3: 291–305.

Williams, G. and Popay, J. (1994) 'Researching the people's health: dilemmas and opportunities for social scientists', in J. Popay and G. Williams (eds) *Researching the People's Health*, London: Routledge.

Witherow, J. (1996) *Change Your Life: A Six-Part Guide to Health and Diet*, London: *The Sunday Times* and PPP Healthcare, 7 January.

Chapter 12

Popular health, advanced liberalism and *Good Housekeeping* magazine

Robin Bunton

The doctor put my wife on Bengers

Mr A.P., of Breaston, Derby says: – 'Very helpful and a splendid night-cap. My Wife . . . has been down with Pleurisy and the doctor has put her on Bengers, which she finds very helpful. It certainly is all you claim for it and a splendid night-cap.'

Why is Bengers so specially good for you, when you're ill, convalescing, or just not feeling or sleeping too well? Because Bengers is the *only* drink which gives you strengthening nourishment without straining your weakened digestion.

(*Good Housekeeping*, March 1959: 19–20)

You can tell he's a Flora man

Today's man cares. He looks after himself. He cares about what he eats. Flora is part of healthy eating. That's why you find more men becoming Flora men. Their wives know they like that light, delicate taste. And Flora is made with pure sunflower oil, so it's high in polyunsaturates. Higher, in fact, than any other nationally available spread. Is there a Flora man in your home?

(*Good Housekeeping*, June 1980: 264)

The two quotes above are the texts of advertisements appearing in *Good Housekeeping* magazine. Only twenty-one years apart, they represent two different rationalities of health care and two different strategies of governance. The first ad appeals to a relatively unproblematic medical authority and presents the qualities of a health-enhancing product to a relatively docile subject preparing to care for his family. The second ad (which also shows a man taking exercise) appeals to a generalised scientific knowledge and promotes the product as a signifier of a whole lifestyle to an active subject who is enterprising and self-caring. In this chapter I want to address the difference between these two health care regimes, drawing on Michel Foucault's work, and to suggest that the study of magazines and popular health is a useful vantage point for such analysis. As illustration I draw on a study of health representations in *Good Housekeeping* magazine since 1959.

FOUCAULT AND THE ANALYSIS OF CONTEMPORARY HEALTH CARE

Foucault's work has had a continuing effect on the study of health and medicine and yet most of his key texts drawn upon by medical sociologists and others were written prior to a number of major transformations in most Western health care regimes, in particular those involving economic restructuring, increased use of the market mechanisms in the organisation and delivery of health care, an appeal to consumer choice, and a devaluing of state intervention. These changes may be described as the onset of advanced liberal rationalities of the governance of health and welfare. In this chapter I argue that Foucault's work continues to provide insight and focus to the study of a health care system in transition and one profoundly immersed in consumer culture.

Perhaps the main contribution of Foucault to the study of health and illness has been through his analysis of the relationships between certain discourses, the body and the exercise of power. His work on the clinic, the asylum and sexuality in particular examines power/knowledge at work on the individual body and on populations of bodies. A sociology of health and illness has gained much from this 'powerful framework for the development of a theoretical medical sociology addressed to the central issues of meaning, structure, social order and power' (Turner 1995: 11). Foucault's history of the present has more often dealt with medicine and health tangentially, as part of other projects. The concern was, as Foucault himself notes, for 'the different ways in our culture that humans develop knowledge about themselves' (1988: 17). Whilst these analyses are fundamental to our understanding of the present, and continue to have a relevance for contemporary analysis, they do not specifically address a number of more recent developments in health relating to the restructuring of health care systems under 'New Right' led governments, developments in the structure of medical knowledge and the emergence of recent epidemics, particularly HIV/AIDS. To address these issues we need to turn to Foucault's more general observations on neo-liberalism and the work of others, inspired by Foucault's work, dealing specifically with features of contemporary health and social care.

Nikolas Rose has undertaken a number of studies drawing on Foucault's notion of governmentality which extend from the government of oneself to the collective government of souls: the government of households as well as the arts of the government practised by a prince (Foucault 1991) or what has been termed 'the conduct of conduct' (Burchell 1993). Foucault's accounts of Western neo-liberal thought in post-war years examined fundamental challenges to the idea of the welfare state (Gordon 1991). Rose has developed this analysis distinguishing between liberalism and what he refers to as 'advanced liberalism', which can usefully be applied to contemporary health care (Rose 1993). Liberalism, for Rose, seen as a *formula of rule* has four significant features. First, liberalism inaugurated a new relation between government and knowledge, a new mode of authority, which tied government to positive knowledges of human conduct. This came about because of the nineteenth-century growth of expertise in the human sciences which was directed at solving a series of problems that made indviduals governable. Second, liberalism depended upon subjects being active in their own government, invested a great deal in the existence of free individuals and sought to shape and regulate that freedom in a social form, specifying what is acceptable 'civilised' behaviour to be rewarded with the rights of citizenship and that which is not, sanctioned by exclusion. Third, liberalism sought to utilise and instrumentalise forms of authority and expertise outside the state apparatus to govern, harnessing professional authority through various forms of licensing and through bureaucratisation. The emergence of this relationship between state and expertise was not systematically conceived but the outcome of responses to various *ad hoc* emerging disturbances such as epidemics, crime, pauperism, insanity and other issues labelled as 'social problems'. Finally, liberalism's rationality involved a continual questioning of the activity of rule itself. It was not so much a formula of rule as a constant suspicion of rule. It is these features of liberalism which can be recognised in the emergence of the 'welfare state' in the nineteenth and twentieth centuries, characterised by Donzelot as the 'socialization of society' (Donzelot 1979). The territory of 'the social' emerged as strategy to resolve a number of fragmentation and individualising processes produced by industrialisation and urbanisation. Social insurance for health and welfare care introduced technologies of government by which governments could guarantee the freedoms of the individual and of capital whilst simultaneously harnessing the role of professionals and their authority (Rose 1993: 293).

Advanced liberalism by contrast, Rose argues, as it developed in Germany in the post-war period and in the Anglo-Saxon world, has three different features. First, it engenders a new relationship between expertise and politics. Rather than totally respecting sources of expertise on human conduct, it penetrates these with a series of new techniques for exercising critical scrutiny and budgetary discipline, including accountancy and audit. Calculative regimes and financial management have entered the relationship between professional and the state. Audit and marketisation has rendered expertise governable by eradicating the uncertainty of truth claims. An apparent devolution of power is achieved by handing over decisions to consumers.

Second, advanced liberalism involves a pluralisation of technologies. Social technologies of the welfare state are reconfigured and detached from centralised regulating technologies in favour of various autonomised agencies. This has involved supplanting the norms of service and dedication with those of competition and customer demand. Finally, advanced liberalism involves a new specification of the subject of government in which the client becomes a customer and risk management is privatised. O'Malley (1992) has described increased ways in which citizens are obliged to adopt a calculative and 'prudent' personal relationship to risk and danger. Social work or physician-based care gives way to the self-help group and the help-line, and citizens take on a new authority of their own. Power effects under this style of governance are different to those experienced under liberalism. People do not possess or seize power and power cannot be calculated as a 'zero sum', as modern citizens are largely agents of their own government (Rose 1989).

We can usefully apply this analysis of advanced liberalism to contemporary restructured health care systems. Three features in these changes roughly correspond to Rose's schema: the privileging of the market mechanism in regulating medical practice, a pluralisation of technologies of health care involving a shift in the temporal and spatial organisation of health care, and an increased emphasis on individual, community and commercial sector responsibility for health status.

The first of these involves the increased use of the market principle to organise and distribute services and to regulate expertise in the delivery of health care. In the UK the introduction of the market was led by 'New Right' thinking of Conservative administrations. *The*

Griffiths Report (DHSS 1983), typical of this thinking, represented a significant move away from a largely consensus-led approach involving teams of doctors, nurses and administrators, towards a system of commercial business management borrowed from the commercial sector which turned administrators into business managers (Cox 1991; Harrison *et al.* 1990; Hunter 1991). The introduction of the principles of an 'internal market' into the NHS, with a separation between the purchasers and providers and increased use of private contractors in health care delivery, has been seen as a major threat to clinical autonomy and the system of professional dominance (Gabe *et al.* 1994). In primary care the delegation of budgetary control to general practitioners and the imposition of new GP contracts and a mechanism of audit and management of services by the Family Practitioner Service Authorities has led to increased commercialisation of the sector overall whilst introducing elements of autonomy for GPs (Butland 1993).

As well as constituting a 'New Right' challenge to medical dominance and an attempt to eradicate 'dependency' culture, these changes also realigned professional and political strategies. Osborne (1993: 355), analysing medicine as government, argues that such changes to the UK health care system did not fundamentally erode professional power, but merely introduced a 'novel form of medical government' which allows the medical field to be both governed and self-governing. Physicians were set to work alongside managers to align clinical 'truth' with economic rationality.

A second significant change in Western and Antipodean health care systems has been a noticeable pluralisation in health intervention technologies and a shift in the temporal and spatial location of care. Evidence for this shift comes from a number of quarters and is nicely encapsulated in the title of the UK government's policy document of the mid-1970s – *Prevention and Health: Everybody's Business* (DHSS 1976). It was around this time that a series of policy statements emerged redefining the responsibilities of governments towards health care. The influential Canadian Ministerial report by Lalonde (1974) directed attention to the influences over health far beyond the reaches of government and the provision of health care – the environment, lifestyle and the bio-structure. WHO programmes at that time were working to develop strategies to respond to the 'new social, political, economic and environmental challenges' facing nation states by redesigning health policy and health infrastructures (WHO 1991). Health promotion introduced an expanded agenda and a range of new sites in which to intervene to promote health, including the public policy arena, the environment, the community (WHO 1986). Health was now an issue of intersectoral collaboration and personal skill development and required an attempt to reorient the health service. Health for All 2000, perhaps the best-known of WHO initiatives (Davies and Kelly 1993), has attempted to identify new sites of concern – healthy cities, healthy schools and healthy workplaces.

Castel, echoing Foucault's concerns with the 'dangerous individual' (Foucault 1988), has suggested that we can conceptualise a transformation that has moved from a health (and social) care regime based upon 'dangerousness' to one based upon 'risk' (Castel 1991). The new strategies involve dissolving the notion of a subject or a concrete individual and replacing it with a combination of *factors* of risk. Interventions essentially are no longer a matter of face-to-face contact between the professional and client. Rather, the concern of the professional is for the *flow of populations* and a range of abstract factors deemed liable to produce risk in general. The shift from a system of care for the ill is transformed into a system for monitoring the health and welfare of populations. Epidemiological survey data under the regime of risk becomes the main strategy of the health professional and the dispensary becomes the focus of a new, extended medical gaze (Armstrong 1983). New modes of surveillance, aided by technological advances, make the calculation of probabilities of 'systematic pre-detection' more and more sophisticated. Populations are increasingly being managed on the basis of their profiles in relation to factors such as their age, social class, occupation, gender, relationships, locality, lifestyle and consumption, and interventions take more diverse forms.

Risk management has entered more consciously into government policy statements on health such as that made in the UK's *Health of the Nation* document (DH 1992a), which has drawn heavily upon international health promotion discourse in constructing a strategy on risk. In this statement, and supporting documentation, it stresses population and risk, claiming: 'Two basic approaches can be taken to the promotion of good health, the population approach and the high-risk approach. The most effective programme combines both approaches' (DH 1992b: 33). This document outlines risk factor targets such as the reduction in cigarette smoking, saturated fatty acid intake and the number of people who are obese.

Health risk discourse has become dominant in the study of social aspects of health and public health, and health promotion in particular, and has received some critical attention in recent years, particularly with reference to its regulatory potential (Baum 1993; Bunton 1990, 1992; Gillick 1984; Green 1995; Greco 1993; Lupton 1995; Nettleton and Bunton 1995; Petersen 1996; Petersen and Lupton 1996; Stevenson and Burke 1991). Several chapters in this volume also refer to such developments. The regulation of risk allows population strategies but also individualising focuses. Although a collective concept (Ewald 1991), in health promotion discourse risk has been made 'internal' and an individual quality. This contrasts with the 'external', environmental risk highlighted in the work of Beck and Douglas (Lupton 1995). 'Risk-takers' become demonised as the new 'sinners' of a secular discourse which has replaced religious belief systems (Douglas and Wildavsky 1982), such as those who smoke in public, drink and drive, or practise unsafe sex. Forms of group identification, exclusion, marginalisation and regulation are practised, defining some as 'at risk', some as 'Self' and some as 'Other' (Figlio 1989). Drug 'scares' are a good example of the use of risk in this way. 'Chinamen' were made 'Other' during the cocaine scare of the early twentieth century (Kohn 1992) in a similar way that black youths have been marginalised in more recent anti-drug campaigns in the USA (Reaves and Campbell 1994). Risk profiling and management, then, are strategies that can be analysed using Foucault's problematisations of expertise and scientific discourse under a general interest in governmentality, as Petersen's chapter outlines above. Risk management also applies to processes of individual governance and management of the self, and can apply to a third significant change in health care systems – the privatisation of health care and individual risk management.

Contemporary risk profiling and the rational calculation of personal conduct have received critical attention in a number of quarters. Giddens has made much of the monitoring and management of the self as a project as a feature of reflexive modernisation (Giddens 1991). Modernity, he argues, confronts the individual with complex and diverse choices as a result of the entry of global and abstract systems into more and more daily concerns. Social relationships are increasingly lifted out from the immediacy of tradition or *Gemeinschaft* and rearticulated in other times and spaces. Expert systems, such as medicine, provide a means of judgement that outstrip and supersede relationships based upon trust. Everyday life becomes saturated with expert knowledge that advises us what food to eat, what exercise to take, from routine health education through to more in-depth therapy. Self-realisation takes place through more reflexive consideration of lifestyle options and *life-planning*. It is only under such conditions that the 'search for self-identity' becomes understandable. The self is seen here as a project or a narrative that has to be constantly rewritten. Self-actualisation is understood in terms of a balance between opportunity and risk.

Through risk profiling individuals construct enterprising, calculating and prudent selves appropriate to advanced liberal rationality (Petersen in chapter 10; Petersen 1996; Rose 1993). Subjectivity is accomplished through such discourse and health becomes, at least in part, the responsibility of citizens. It is in recognition of this phenomenon that accusations of 'healthism' (Crawford 1980) and 'bodyism' (Dutton 1995) have emerged. The pursuit of the ideals of health, fitness, youthfulness and beauty occurs as a particular moral form. Gillick (1984) has pointed out that the incentives for such self-care have come from a number of quarters including sport, leisure industries and a more general economic rationale. The emergence of employee assistance programmes, stress management courses and reduced insurance premiums for those with healthier lifestyles are clear examples of this encouragement.

Self-care and self-help have long since run alongside medical expertise, often in response to discontent and scepticism regarding the efficacy of professional medicine (Kickbusch 1989). Coupled with a rise in consumerism, the self-help movement has had some policy recognition in the UK recently with the introduction of the *Patient's Charter* (DH 1991). These developments have been seen by some as a challenge to modern medicine (Kelleher *et al.* 1994). Considered from the perspective of advanced liberal governance, such phenomena appear ideal strategies for producing the enterprising, healthy citizen. Rather than challenging medicine, they are integral to liberalism's own self-questioning of the right to govern, which incites active citizenship.

In summary, I have been arguing that we can conceive of a number of recent changes in health care as echoing features of transformations in governmental techniques and rationality associated with advanced liberalism. These features have been analytically separated here, though in fact are likely to interact or be seen to act simultaneously in a number of sites. For example, the introduction of the market into health care has affected not simply the nature of knowledge and the regulation of professional practice but also the nature of self-help and self-care in the form of commodification of health. In contemporary consumer culture, health, identity and consumption are inextricably entwined (a point that will be explored on p. 235). Equally, we cannot easily separate the techniques for regulating the health of populations from those used in constructing healthy subjects. Today concern for health is not restricted to a particular time and place as described in Parsons's account of the sick role (Parsons 1951). Health is increasingly de-differentiated: it has become integral to the management of the various parts of our lives.

These changes have a number of implications for the power effects within contemporary health care and for the type of analyses we can make of them. They also suggest new sites for analysis. Whereas much of previous Foucauldian sociology and history of health and medicine has focused on expert discourses, the sites of health regimes characteristic of advanced liberalism are likely to be more dispersed.

In the remainder of this chapter I want to explore one such site: popular health as found in women's magazines. This analysis will draw upon and extend the analyses put forward so far and evaluate their durability for contemporary analyses of health care.

MAGAZINES AND POPULAR HEALTH

It is Foucault's earlier work focusing upon expert discourses that has received most attention in the sociology of health and illness, probably because it could be used to support a critique of professional power, as Armstrong's and Lupton's chapters above illustrate. By contrast, other forms of discourse, which featured in Foucault's later work, such as everyday knowledge and popular forms of knowledge, have received less attention in Foucauldian-inspired work. This neglect has left more detailed and useful analyses of power/knowledge of other sites, such as popular culture and everyday discourse and practice, relatively underdeveloped. It has meant, for example, a neglect of certain mundane yet important aspects of life that span expert systems on the one hand and everyday knowledge and practice on the other. Valverde (1996) has shown how 'habits' have a governing potential that falls neither into the realm of discipline nor the realm of pastoral care – the Christian regime that preceded disciplinary power. This drawback is particularly apparent in relation to contemporary health, and health promotion in particular, where there has been an increased propensity for expert knowledge to be dispersed and concerns for health to be extended to an infinitely broader focus on 'well-being' (O'Brian 1995). There would appear to be a tendency in the sociology of health and illness to reproduce a general assumption in Western (and modern) cultures that expert knowledges are distinct from 'lay' knowledges requiring distinct forms of study (Calnan 1987; Davison *et al.* 1991; Williams and Popay 1994). The boundary between lay and expert knowledge is in fact far less clear than can be assumed from such studies. Here I am concerned with an area that falls within the increasingly blurred boundaries between lay and expert health knowledge reproduced in magazines.

Magazines and the media are sites of increasing importance to contemporary problematisations of health. On the one hand there is an increased propensity found in magazines and periodicals to report on health matters and become involved in health education (Black 1995; Elliot 1994). On the other hand, there has arisen a field of expertise in health communications which has focused on the ability of campaigns and advertising to promote or diminish healthy behaviours and lifestyles (Irwin 1989; Petersen 1994; Bunton et al. 1991). Coming to prominence in the age of capitalist mass production, magazines are not only commodities themselves but also important means of commodification and product promotion (Beetham 1996). In an attempt to turn to the field of 'popular health' and to explore aspects of contemporary governance under advanced liberalism I will draw upon a study of representations of health in four years of Good Housekeeping magazine: 1959, 1976, 1980 and 1994/5.[1] One aim of this study was to document the development of health and consumer culture in the post-war period. There are a number of reasons for anticipating increased growth in health-related consumer culture over this period linked to a more general privileging of bodily appearance, youthfulness, vitality, health and beauty and the 'aestheticisation' of everyday life associated with consumer culture (Bunton and Burrows 1995; Featherstone 1991; Glassner 1995, 1992; Lupton 1995). Analysis of Good Housekeeping magazine found an almost threefold increase in health-related articles and advertisements between 1959 and 1994/5 and significant changes in the style of health coverage. In the remainder of this chapter I examine three themes relating to representations of health under advanced liberalism: changes in the nature of popular health knowledge, commodification of health products, and the fabrication of the caring self in magazine readers.

MAGAZINE MEDICINE

Magazine knowledge is popular health knowledge that lies beyond the professional epicentre of medical authority, yet it reports and comments upon medical findings, extrapolates and interprets these findings for the general reader and makes judgements about the quality of that knowledge. As interpreters of health knowledge, magazine writers and editors play an active role in what has been referred to as a 'politics of health information' (Farrant and Russell 1986). *Good Housekeeping* magazine acts as a vantage point on medicine. It carries authority related to its representations of expert knowledge and also to its warrant as a 'quality' magazine. Magazine medicine, then, spans and often bridges specialist and non-specialist knowledge systems, or what Ludwick Fleck describes as inner, 'esoteric' knowledge at the centre of disciplines and an outer, 'exotic' circle (Fleck 1979). Exotic knowledge consists of the 'educated amateur's' or popular knowledge and is characterised by a certain simplicity and vividness concerning the nature of the world. This knowledge, he notes, has a tendency to lack detail and controversy. 'Inner' science on the other hand is produced by and for the expert and offers more versions of science; it is more provisional, tentative and less certain. Fleck refers also to 'journal science' which is to some extent experimental and attempts to 'discover' or create knowledge; it defies organisation into a unified whole and is inherently contradictory, incongruous and fragmented. This distinction is a useful one to bear in mind when considering magazine or popular knowledge.

Several changes occurred in *Good Housekeeping*'s representation of medical authority since 1959. The first of these may be described as the 'disappearance of the doctor'.[2] Whilst medical articles explicitly drawing upon medical authority were present in 1959, new forms of medical reporting appeared from 1976 to 1995. Doctor's pages appeared, for example, either in the form of a letter written by a doctor, or a round-up of medical research by a doctor. A page titled 'Medicine in the news', for example, includes an article billed as 'Dr Susan Garth looks at some of the research and developing techniques that may help us all to better health'. Other articles appeared in a section called 'Family centre'. The doctor's authority is demonstrated by the reporting of anecdotes from the surgery and knowledge of latest research as well as reassuring advice given on topics such as treatment for the deaf, influenza vaccines, morning sickness, hair care, cigarettes and cancer, school children's health, and counsel against 'old wives' tales'. Very few feature articles relating to health appeared in 1959, the drama of a 'hole in the heart' miracle operation being the exception. This story of heroic medicine supported the bio-medical order of the advice columns.

By 1980 doctors' columns were much depleted and they had completely disappeared by 1994/5. In contemporary articles the reader is spoken to directly by the magazine, which gives 'the facts', often quoting the source: the *British Medical Journal*, *The Lancet*, etc. There is now no intermediary between the knowledge and the reader, except occasionally a named reporter with no medical qualification. Medical knowledge is reported in its own regular section titled simply 'Health' – an apparent shift towards prevention. In contemporary articles, not only are doctors absent, but *Good Housekeeping* increasingly carries articles which are critical of medical authority, including titles such as: 'Escape the tranquilliser trap', 'Borderline smear' (what to do in the light of medical advice), 'Children in hospital', 'Are these the best GPs in Britain?' Alongside such articles, a new section appeared by the 1990s called 'Mind and body: complementary treatments reviewed'. This section invites the reader to consider and take up different complementary medicines. Contrary to advice in 1959, traditional remedies are cultivated and information from a whole range of medicines/therapies is presented. In this case then, contrary to Fleck's observations, current popular knowledge in *Good Housekeeping* is seemingly highly controversial and represents and embraces contradiction.

That medical knowledge is not unproblematically accepted by the general population is well documented and recent accounts of health knowledge have increasingly highlighted resistance to the grand narrative of professionally dominated medicine. Williams and Popay (1994) provide an account of a local challenge to a medical account of the dumping of toxic waste into drinking water. Fox also takes up the notion of the relativisation of medical knowledge and increasing competition to medicine from other forms of knowledge (Fox 1991). The new discourses on health promotion have been argued to provide further instances of resistance to the grand narrative of bio-medicine, particularly where projects actively seek to integrate the voice of 'others' into health programmes (Kelly and Charlton 1995). We might see the changes in *Good Housekeeping* magazine as signs of a broader blurring of boundaries between esoteric and exotic circles of medical knowledge, and perhaps also a pluralisation of technologies of governance Rose associates with advanced liberalism.

Turner has analysed a somewhat similar pluralisation active in the medical curriculum (1992a). Market-led Research and Development commissioning, he argues, has been successful in engendering interdisciplinary cooperation by introducing competitive pressure and a deregulated academic market place which has made collaboration a necessity. He points out that such a developments raise fundamental questions for medical authority. The commercialisation of medicine undermines the idealism of the Hippocratic tradition (Starr 1982) just as commercialisation of intellectual life raises questions about the traditional institutions of professional knowledge (Bauman 1988). The implications for medicine are profound:

> If deregulation and postmodern epistemologies are both effects of changes in consumption, economic production and advanced technology, then we may expect the hierarchical division between scientific medicine and alternative medicine (like the distinction between high culture and mass culture) to collapse as the traditional autonomy of the medical profession is eroded through the invasion of corporations into the health market.
>
> (Turner 1992a: 145)

The implication of this analysis is that, just as for Lyotard (1984) the knowledge system was transformed by the advent of post-industrial society, with an emphasis on communications revolution, cybernetics, the growth of the internet and associated dominance of the service sector, medicine will be transformed and previously professionally protected knowledge boundaries will be breached. The medical curriculum as well as preventive health will be reduced in a crude commodification or a process of 'McDonaldisation'. If shifts in the organisation of medical knowledge described here are at all representative, then they might be explained from the perspective of analysis of new forms of governance and the onset of advanced liberalism. More diverse and dispersed knowledge systems may be called upon to support more flexible interventions in 'health care' and aligned with economic rationality. Analysis of health commodities illustrate best, perhaps, the alignment of health knowledge and market rationality. There would appear to be increased potential for products to act as communicators of health messages and thereby function as carriers of disciplinary knowledge.

HEALTH COMMODITIES

Studies of consumption have stressed the ways in which an expansion in commodity production has had a profound effect upon the cultural sphere and generated new cultural forms and new forms of identity (Featherstone 1991). In the health sphere the growth in 'health-related' goods and services is influenced by a market logic which produces both new products and new, more discerning, health-conscious consumers. This can be seen in *Good Housekeeping*'s growth in health consumer products. The list of health products advertised in one issue of *Good Housekeeping* in 1959 typically included, for example: laxatives, slimming aids, anti-rheumatic products, cough medicine, men's surgical support and various 'healthy' cleaning products (e.g. Jeye's toilet tissue). By 1994/5 these had been supplemented by a number of additional products such that a typical issue might advertise: low-fat spread, a variety of vitamins, fruit juice, Kellog's Bran Flakes, anti-diarrhoea products, *Health and Beauty* magazine, water filters, trainers, sugar substitutes and Volvo (safe) cars. In the intervening years there had been a significant 'transvaluing' of products (Featherstone 1991). Certain products' original use-values had become increasingly articulated in terms of health, e.g. margarine and Volvo cars. At stake in this expansion is more than a simple expansion in the market. The value of these products has shifted far beyond the product itself to incorporate elements of 'lifestyle' and social distinction (Leiss 1983).

Health products between the late 1950s and 1995 took on an expressive as well as an instrumental function. As well as rationally calculating their need for trainers, track suits, pure spring water or low-fat spread, consumers were encouraged to consider the expressive quality of these products and what they said about their identity. Products became, in Leiss's term, 'positional goods'. Bourdieu has pointed to the ways such products can become integral to a system of classification and social distinction (1984) and a part of the *habitus* of a class or social group. There would appear to have been a shift from more specifically ascetic health product consumption towards a consumption which stressed 'self-expression', included self-formation and indicated group affiliation. A class of consumer was being formed that appreciated healthy diets, staying in shape and increasing body potential. Health-related patterns of consumption can be analysed for their social meaning with reference to this patterning. Examining British middle-class patterns of consumption, Savage *et al.* (1992: 99–158) found an association between high income and consumption of health and body maintenance products, though also an excess and indulgence in eating and drinking by higher income groups (Bunton and Burrows 1995). The creation and maintenance or 'policing' of such product positioning is undertaken by what Bourdieu has referred to as the 'new cultural intermediaries' (Bourdieu 1984). For certain health products, expressive consumption value was being carefully con-structed by product design. This is illustrated by the rise of new 'soft' toilet tissue products.

In 1959 cleanliness products were amongst only a few products to make explicit claim to health value. We might see this as a coding of health by reference to 'germ theory' or contagion. One product, Bronco toilet tissue, professed: 'It's a healthy sign when Bronco's in the house.'

The safest tissue

Medical opinion says that to avoid infection toilet tissue should be non-absorbent, Bronco is as non-absorbent as toilet tissue can be made, possessing only that degree of absorbency which is absolutely necessary – that's why doctors recommend it.

(*Good Housekeeping* February 1959: 127)

The advent of 'soft' toilet tissue represented a departure from a health and cleanliness coding by stressing the luxuriousness of the product. Coincidentally, we have some access to the rationale of the 'cultural intermediaries' concerned with developing this product. Miller and Rose (1996) have examined the work of the Tavistock Institute of Human Relations (TIHR) in market research and product design in the 1950s. The alliance of 'psy' expertise with that of the commercial sector exemplifies new ways of governing the acts of consumption. Regional surveys were undertaken on this product to ascertain the social and psychological significance of toilet tissue. It was established that health, cleanliness and reliability were associated with 'hard' tissue and that, conversely, some anxiety about reliability with vigorous use was linked to the new 'soft' product, as well as some unease about the association of pleasure with this commodity. The TIHR were able to endorse the new product despite protestations against softness. The TIHR concluded that upward class mobility aspirations demanded that emphasis on 'extra' pleasures should be placed on products, including aesthetic pleasure or social satisfaction. It was, as Miller and Rose point out, the 'extraneous, or non-functional aspects of products' that were becoming increasingly valued, leading to a 'more permissive and tolerant attitude to pleasurable experiences in general, and especially to pleasure arising from care of the body or from natural bodily functions' (TIHR 1956: 2).

This detailed analysis of signifying strategies in relation to toilet tissue illustrates how health and social value were carefully monitored by cultural intermediaries at the design stage. The new soft toilet tissue made a claim to a new market niche by creating a social distinction. However, this gave traditional 'hard' toilet tissue product's promoters greater opportunities to stress the solid health value of their own products, the value of one product thereby determining that of another. The new product, on TIHR advice, stressed its smooth yet safe qualities and its advantages in reducing the tedium of undertaking personal, family and household tasks. This detailed analysis also reveals the ways in which product design creates desire in consumers, achieved, as Miller and Rose note, not as a simple imposition or by treating the consumers as cultural dopes, but by affording subjects spaces in which to engage in expression and reasoned choice. The construction of consumers was treated as highly problematic and involved a careful combined analysis of the psy-complex, the social group, the product and the study of everyday life (Miller and Rose 1996).

By positioning themselves and consumers, products carry disciplinary signs and disperse technologies of the self. Consumption of goods also involves, as Baudrillard has pointed out, the consumption of a relationship and a sign (1988) – consumption of a set of relationships particular to advanced liberal health, and consumption of the signs of 'good health'. The production and consumption of such positional health goods marries discipline, happiness and profit, illustrated in this case by a product closely related to the care of the self.

CARE OF THE SELF

Perhaps the most obvious application of Foucault's observations on health and the body for the study of 'magazine health' concerns his notion of the 'care of the self'. Petersen notes that there are striking similarities between the processes of self-formation in contemporary culture and the practices of self-care in ancient Greece (Petersen 1994). (Although Foucault has cautioned against assuming that agency has a general form. Problematising conduct and relating it to inner, ethical self-scrutiny and self-control are a dominant feature of Western techniques of living but are by no means universal.) We can note here that a rational, health-promoting self appears to have emerged in 'official discourse' and in magazines' health cultures, stressing enterprise, body work and self-improvement. Contemporary self-health techniques share much with the self-control achieved by body regimen in ancient Greece and, similarly, demonstrate one's ethical worth (Foucault 1985). Common to both periods is a focus on the body and an assumption that a healthy body is the outcome of the actions of a rational subject. The increased importance of preventive health and health communications in contemporary health care regimes suggests a further privileging of the reasoned subject. There may be reason to assume that health in magazines and in the media has more of a propensity to construct the rational subject than other health discourses, as Greco notes (1993). Interaction with the new medical authority of *Good Housekeeping* magazine does not takes place in the emotionally charged consultation. The media cannot engage in other 'curative' forms of medicine but focus instead on prevention and the reasoning, reading, autonomous subject.

On the face of it then, popular health in magazines would seem to be an ideal location from which to observe the positioning of the contemporary subject of health discourses and the acquisition of the techniques for fabricating the healthy self. This approach, which has become common in cultural studies, could be applied to the contemporary subject of health advice and advertisements (Bonney and Wilson 1990). Even a cursory analysis of *Good Housekeeping* suggests that significant re-positioning of the subject of health has taken place. The subject of 1959 discourse was very much the docile body of the 'sick man/woman' (Jewson 1976) of the medical gaze. The subject is the passive receiver of medical advice from doctors or the purchaser of a limited set of goods that are designed to care for individual and family health and cleanliness.

In 1959 advertisements tend to position the consumer in relation to the family. The 'Bengers' food supplement ad illustrates this well. The food supplements market in *Good Housekeeping* targeted the elderly. Another product, 'Complan', shows an elderly couple and runs a banner 'Now you have only each other to care for, you can do it properly. Complan helps you help the ones you love' (*Good Housekeeping* February 1977: 212). The subjects of a great number of other products were the caring, responsible mother, the agent of family health documented in other studies of family health care of the time (Armstrong 1983; Nettleton 1991). By the 1980s and 1990s *Good Housekeeping* had begun to privilege another more independent consumer and the 'narcissistic' reader became a feature of health sections of the magazine. The Flora ad above represents an ad that is family- and lifestyle-oriented yet also narcissistic. It advocates self-care in 'today's caring man'. He cares but is also cared for, supported in his struggle for healthy subjectivity by his similarly caring wife. Flora man (and his wife) is concerned with staying 'in shape', looking after his (and her) body by exercise and acting preventively and positively to promote his (and her) own health. The essence of this contemporary self has been captured in Glassner's description of the 'postmodern self' (Glassner 1989). Giddens's analysis of individual risk profiling and management captures something of the self-positioning in such ads (Giddens 1991, 1992).

Such positioning gives us insight into the techniques of the self engendered by contemporary health promotion in popular representations of health. The enterprising selves portrayed in these advertisements and health columns should not be considered as impositions, however. Foucault was at pains to avoid a simplistic rendering of processes of the formation of subjects. There is a sense in which Foucault's later work acknowledges a self that is autonomous and able to extricate itself from normalising judgements and disciplinary practices (Schrift 1995). More recently, cultural studies has also moved away from a perspective of the 'dominant ideology' and become concerned for the ways in which audiences interpret, select and receive media messages; though, as Petersen notes (1994), there is still much to be done in analysing how different audiences negotiate, identify with, reject and subvert subject positioning. Magazines may be especially interesting in this respect given their open nature and the particular way in which reading of them is practised.

Margaret Beetham (1996) has argued that the periodical or magazine is characterised by a radical heterogeneity and a refusal of a single authorial voice. (Hence some TV and radio programmes describe themselves as such – as a 'mix'.) Most successful magazines will be heterogeneous and include narratives, poems, pictures, competitions and jokes. Magazines are also self-consciously highly temporal – weekly, monthly or quarterly. Their temporary quality gives them an even more open-ended and fluid quality and requires them to be read in a less intense manner than, say, a book or an academic journal. Moreover, they are not a single entity in themselves. Hermes (1995), using Geertz's term, refers to magazines as a 'blurred genre', and identifies three women's magazine types distinguished by readers: traditional, feminist and gossip magazines. She documents how their readers read magazines differently. Such studies undermine notions of the simplistic communication of governing images of health or gender. Given the diversity of forms and the manner in which they are read, these texts are unlikely to position a single reader or even an identifiable 'Good Housekeeper' or 'Cosmo Girl'. Rather we might envisage techniques of the self as being more fragmentary and dispersed. Moreover, we are more likely to find the meaning of the magazines through analysis of the context of reading and browsing. A simple analysis of the processing of a singular subject would seem inappropriate here. We cannot privilege these texts over other discourses and cannot easily draw conclusions concerning the 'readings' and subject positions within them. A more productive strategy would be to draw more broadly upon analysis of reading and identity formation, examining the processes in more detail. Examples of such approaches may be found in feminist critical debate concerning reading 'as women' (Fuss 1989; Mills 1994). This approach would probably preclude an over-rational view of the subject of this new discourse.

Although a full analysis cannot be illustrated here, we can note that *Good Housekeeping* mixes texts and styles in the subjectification of health. Whilst Flora men and women are positioned, so too are independent new women who are able to explore their inner potential for health and self-development. Domestic subjectivity is run alongside self-development discourse and the reader would appear to be left to pick and mix. Given this collage of healthy selves we might identify a more complex problematisation of subjectification, and perhaps one specific to advanced liberalism. This self would have more in common with that associated with the 'postmodern' subject in which coherence and unity give way to 'active stylisation and exploration, transitory experience and surface aesthetic effects' (Featherstone 1991: 95). This problematic is possibly more appropriate to the study of a subject that is both autonomous and disciplined. It might also escape those accounts that would over-rationalise human agency.

SUMMARY

In considering some recent developments in Western health care as features of what Rose has termed 'advanced liberal rationality' I have argued that contemporary medical expertise has increasingly been subject to a marketisation, that health regimes have developed pluralised technologies and new modes of intervention dependent on risk analysis and population management, and that a new, health-promoting subject has been specified that is active and enterprising in his or her own body maintenance. A feature of this new rationality has been a dispersal of health interventions and new sites that have replaced older institutional practices of health care. One such site is popular health as portrayed in women's magazines. I have attempted to draw upon Foucault's work to account for some of the features of advanced liberal health apparent in the production and consumption of popular health in *Good Housekeeping* magazine. Whilst Foucault's notion of governmentality, and Rose's development of it, have provided the context for this study, this analysis has necessarily drawn upon other fields of study, such as sociology of knowledge and consumption and analyses of texts and readers developed in cultural studies and feminist critical studies.

Popular health as promoted in magazines is an increasingly important feature of the advanced liberal health regime and displays some features of that rationale of governance. Health and well-being have become of increasing concern to *Good Housekeeping* since the 1950s and perhaps indicative of increased individualised concern with health and the body. If under advanced liberalism the relationship between expertise and politics becomes increasingly subject to realignment with rational calculation and the market, then magazines present this process in a radical form. Medical knowledge appears to have become marketed as one amongst many knowledges for consumption within the consumption of popular knowledge. The presentation of medical knowledge shifted between the years 1959 and 1994/5. Increasingly, different versions of medicine appeared and medical authority in the form of the doctor would seem to have been diminished. At the same time new, preventive, 'risk-oriented' knowledge became more apparent and challenges to medical authority became routine. Risk technologies facilitated more varied interventions represented in *Good Housekeeping* by newer, 'alternative' prevention and therapeutic recommendations and an increased commodification of health. This newer commodification is directed at lifestyle and social positioning whilst simultaneously providing the techniques of care of the self and subjectification. Health commodities act as carriers of disciplinary power in this respect. There would appear to have been a shift from ascetic health products towards pleasurable healthy products, mobilising the consumer to health, wealth and well-being (Miller and Rose 1996). The subject positioned in these texts would appear to be rather like those in Giddens's account of late modern individuals (1992) who experience themselves and their bodies, their social world and physical worlds, with increasing reflection and uncertainty, increasingly reliant on, yet at the same time increasingly suspicious of, abstract expert knowledge systems.

Magazines are sites where complex, partial and incomplete readings of health and other discourses takes place, in different contexts. Whilst the subjects of magazine discourse are positioned in increasingly privatised ways in advertisements and articles in *Good Housekeeping* over the last thirty years or so, it is difficult to assess the effects of these texts and the uses that are made of them. The practices of caring for the self and the body inevitably involve aspects of discursive domination but also aspects of resistance. Magazines are clearly one source of techniques of the self. The openness of their texts, however, is a challenge to a focus on governmentality and probably a challenge that requires us to look for tools of analysis beyond those provided by Foucault.

NOTES

1 *Good Housekeeping* was chosen for a number of reasons. First, having been around since the 1880s, this periodical allows a detailed analysis over time. Second, the magazine claimed to serve 'the interests of higher life in the household' (McCracken 1993), and sought to determine 'quality' in household consumerism and homemaking. It has been classified as a 'traditionally oriented magazine' (Hermes 1995). It has run a variety of *Good Housekeeping* 'Seals of Approval' – a limited warranty, covering most products advertised, contributing to its portrayal of wholesomeness. It was one of the few women's magazines to spurn lucrative cigarette advertising at some points in its history. Unlike some of the 'new woman' magazines, *Good Housekeeping* appeals to more traditional, stolid domestic values which, in many ways, make it ideal for an examination of the impact of consumer culture on health and other topics. If a new type of problematisation of health has reached the 'heights' of quality magazines, then it would almost certainly be apparent in other popular health sites.

The methodology pursued was a version of what has been termed the 'post-structuralist, semiotic analysis' model, as opposed to 'interactionist' or 'content and narrative' analysis of texts (Manning and Cullum-Swan 1994). This approach consisted of examining, coding and categorising texts for themes, meanings and underlying perspectives. The data collected here are not intended to be representative of magazines of this period but to illustrate and facilitate explorations and examination of some textual themes.

2 Here I am echoing Jewson's observations on the disappearance of the 'sick man' in medical cosmology (Jewson 1976). A similar process would appear to be apparent in the texts of *Good Housekeeping*. There were signs that biomedicine was losing something of its singular authority, exemplified by the disappearance of the sick man's opposite – the doctor.

REFERENCES

Armstrong, D. (1983) *Political Anatomy of the Body: Medical Knowledge in Britain in the Twentieth Century*, Cambridge: Cambridge University Press.
Baudrillard, J. (1988) 'The system of objects', in M. Poster (ed.) *Jean Baudrillard: Selected Writings*, Cambridge: Polity Press.
Baum, F. (1993) 'Healthy cities and change: social movement or bureaucratic tool?', *Health Promotion International*, 8, 1: 31–40.

Bauman, Z. (1988) 'Is there a postmodern sociology?', *Theory, Culture & Society*, 5: 217–37

Beetham, M. (1996) *A Magazine of Her Own? Domesticity and Desire in the Women's Magazine, 1800–1914*, London: Routledge.

Black, M.E.A. (1995) 'What did popular women's magazines from 1929 to 1949 say about breast cancer?', *Cancer Nursing*, 18, 4: 270–7.

Bonney, B. and Wilson, H. (1990) 'Advertising and the manufacture of difference', in M. Alvarado and J.O. Thompson *The Media Reader*, London: British Film Institute.

Bourdieu, P. (1984) *Distinction: A Social Critique of the Judgement of Taste*, London: Routledge.

Bunton, R. (1990) 'Regulating our favourite drug', in P. Abbott and G. Payne (eds) *New Directions in the Sociology of Health*, London: Falmer.

Bunton, R. (1992) 'More than a woolly jumper: health promotion as social regulation', *Critical Public Health*, 3, 2: 4–11.

Bunton, R. and Burrows, R. (1995) 'Consumption and health in the "epidemiological" clinic of late modern medicine', in R. Bunton, S. Nettleton and R. Burrows (eds) *The Sociology of Health Promotion*, London: Routledge.

Bunton, R., Murphey, S. and Bennett, P. (1991) 'Theories of behavioural change and their use in health promotion', *Health Education Research: Theory and Practice*, 6, 2: 153–62.

Burchell, G. (1993) 'Liberal government and techniques of the self', *Economy and Society*, 22, 3: 267–344.

Butland, G. (1993) 'Commissioning for quality', *British Medical Journal*, 306: 251–2.

Calnan, M. (1987) *Health and Illness: The Lay Perspective*, London: Tavistock.

Castel, R. (1991) 'From dangerousness to risk', in G. Burchell, C. Gordon and P. Miller (eds) *The Foucault Effect: Studies in Governmentality*, London: Harvester Wheatsheaf.

Cox, D. (1991)'Health service management – a sociological view: Griffiths and the non-negotiated order of the hospital', in J. Gabe, M. Calnan and M. Bury (eds) *The Sociology of the Health Service*, London: Routledge.

Crawford, R. (1980) 'Healthism and the medicalization of everyday life', *International Journal of Health Services*, 10, 3: 365–88.

Davies, J. and Kelly, M. (eds) (1993) *Healthy Cities: Research and Practice*, London: Routledge.

Davison, C., Davey-Smith, G. and Frankel, S. (1991) 'Lay epidemiology and the prevention paradox: the implications of coronary candidacy for health education', *Sociology of Health & Illness*, 13, 1: 1–19.

DH (Department of Health) (1991) *The Patient's Charter*, London: HMSO.

DH (Department of Health) (1992a) *The Health of the Nation: A Strategy for Health in England*, London: HMSO.

DH (Department of Health) (1992b) *The Health of the Nation: Key Area Handbook; Coronary Heart Disease and Stroke*, London: HMSO.

DHSS (Department of Health and Social Security) (1976) *Prevention and Health: Everybody's Business*, London: HMSO.

DHSS (Department of Health and Social Security) (1983) *NHS Management Enquiry (Griffiths Report)*, London: HMSO.

Donzelot, J. (1979) *The Policing of Families*, London: Hutchinson.

Douglas, M. and Calvas, M. (1990) 'The self as risk-taker: a cultural theory of contagion in relation to AIDS', *Sociological Review*, 38, 3: 445–64.

Douglas, M. and Wildavsky, A. (1982) *Risk and Culture*, Oxford: Basil Blackwell.

Dutton, K.R. (1995) *The Perfectible Body: The Western Ideal of Physical Development*, London: Cassell.

Elliot, J.B. (1994) 'A content analysis of the health information provided in women's magazines', *Health Libraries Review*, 11: 96–103.

Ewald, F. (1991) 'Insurance and risk', in G. Burchell, C. Gordon and P. Miller (eds) *The Foucault Effect: Studies in Governmentality*, London: Harvester Wheatsheaf.

Farrant, W. and Russell, J. (1986) *The Politics of Health Information*, London: Health Education Council.

Featherstone, M. (1991) *Consumer Culture and Postmodernism*, London: Sage.

Figlio, C. (1989) 'Unconscious aspects of health and the public sphere', in B. Richards (ed.) *Crisis of the Self: Further Essays on Psychoanalysis and Politics*, London: Free Association Books.

Fleck, L. (1979) *Genesis and Development of a Scientific Fact*, Chicago and London: University of Chicago Press.

Foucault, M. (1985) *The History of Sexuality, Vol. 2: The Use of Pleasure*, New York: Random House.

Foucault, M. (1988) 'The dangerous individual', in L. Kritzman (ed.) *Michel Foucault: Politics, Philosophy, Culture; Interviews and Other Writings*, London: Routledge.

Foucault, M. (1991) 'Governmentality', in G. Burchell, C. Gordon and P. Miller (eds) *The Foucault Effect*, Brighton: Harvester Wheatsheaf.

Fox, N.J. (1991) 'Postmodernism, rationality and the evaluation of health care', *Sociological Review*, 39, 4: 709–44.

Fuss, D. (1989) *Essentially Speaking: Feminism, Nature and Difference*, New York: Routledge.

Gabe, J., Kelleher, D. and Williams, G. (eds) (1994) *Challenging Medicine*, London: Routledge.

Giddens, A. (1991) *Modernity and Self-Identity: Self and Society in the Late Modern Age*, Cambridge: Polity Press.

Giddens, A. (1992) *The Transformation of Intimacy*, Cambridge: Polity Press.

Gillick, M.R. (1984) 'Health promotion, jogging, and the pursuit of the moral life', *Journal of Health, Politics, Policy and Law*, 9, 3: 369–84.

Glassner, B. (1989) 'Fitness and the postmodern self', *Journal of Health and Social Behaviour*, 30: 180–91.

Glassner, B. (1992) *Bodies: The Tyranny of Perfection*, Los Angeles: Lowell House.

Glassner, B. (1995) 'In the name of health', in R. Bunton, S. Nettleton and R. Burrows (eds) *The Sociology of Health Promotion*, London: Routledge.

Gordon, C. (1991) 'Governmental rationality: an introduction', in G. Burchell, C. Gordon and P. Miller (eds) *The Foucault Effect: Studies in Governmentality*, London: Harvester Wheatsheaf.

Greco, M. (1993) 'Psychosomatic subjects and the "duty to be well": personal agency within medical rationality', *Economy and Society*, 22, 3: 357–72.

Green, J. (1995) 'Accidents and the risk society: some problems with prevention', in R. Bunton, S. Nettleton and R. Burrows (eds) *The Sociology of Health Promotion*, New York: Routledge.

Harrison, S., Hunter, D. and Pollitt, C. (1990) *The Dynamics of British Health Policy*, London: Unwin Hyman.

Hermes, J. (1995) *Reading Women's Magazines: An analysis of everyday media use*, Cambridge: Polity Press.

Hunter, D. (1991) 'Managing medicine: a response to "the crisis"', *Social Science and Medicine*, 32: 441–9.

Irwin, H. (1989) 'Health communication: the research agenda', *Media Information Australia*, 54: 32–40.

Jewson, N. (1976) 'The disappearance of the sick man from medical cosmology, 1770–1870', *Sociology*, 10: 225–44.

Kelleher, D., Gabe, J. and Williams, G. (1994) 'Understanding medical dominance in the modern world', in J. Gabe, D. Kelleher and G. Williams (eds) *Challenging Medicine*, London: Routledge.

Kelly, M. and Charlton, B. (1995) 'The modern and the postmodern in health promotion', in R. Bunton, S. Nettleton and R. Burrows (eds) *The Sociology of Health Promotion*, London: Routledge.

Kickbusch, I. (1989) 'Self-care in health promotion', *Social Science and Medicine*, 29: 125–30.

Kohn, M. (1992) *Dope Girls: The Birth of the British Drug Underground*, London: Lawrence and Wishart.

Lalonde, M. (1974) *A New Perspective on the Health of Canadians*, Ottawa: Information Canada.

Leiss, W. (1983) 'The icons of the marketplace', *Theory, Culture & Society*, 1, 3: 24–35.

Lupton, D. (1995) *The Imperative of Health: Public Health and the Regulated Body*, London: Sage.

Lyotard, J.F. (1984) *The Post-Modern Condition: A Report on Knowledge*, trans. G. Bennington and B. Mascum, Manchester: Manchester University Press.

McCracken, E. (1993) *Decoding Women's Magazines*, Basingstoke: Macmillan.

Manning, K. and Cullum-Swan, B. (1994) 'Narrative, content, and semiotic analysis', in N.K. Denzin and Y.S. Lincoln (eds) *Handbook of Qualitative Research*, London: Sage.

Miller, P. and Rose, N. (1996) 'Mobilizing the consumer: assembling the subject of consumption', *Theory, Culture & Society*, 14, 1.

Mills, S. (ed.) (1994) *Gendering the Reader*, Hemel Hempstead: Harvester Wheatsheaf.

Nettleton, S. (1991) 'Wisdom, diligence and teeth: discursive practices and the creation of mothers', *Sociology of Health & Illness*, 13, 1: 98–111.

Nettleton, S. and Bunton, R. (1995) 'Sociological critiques of health promotion', in R. Bunton, S. Nettleton and R. Burrows (eds) *The Sociology of Health Promotion*, New York: Routledge.

O'Brian, M. (1995) 'Health and lifestyle: a critical mess? Notes on the de-differentiation of health', in R. Bunton, S. Nettleton and R. Burrows (eds) *The Sociology of Health Promotion*, New York: Routledge.

O'Malley, P. (1992) 'Risk, power and crime prevention', *Economy and Society*, 21, 3: 252–75.

Osborne, T. (1993) 'On liberalism, neo-liberalism and the "liberal profession" of medicine', *Economy and Society*, 22, 3: 345–56.

Parsons, T. (1951) *The Social System*, Glencoe, Illinois: Free Press.

Petersen, A.R. (1994) 'Governing images: media constructions of the "normal", "healthy" subject', *Media Information Australia*, 72: 32–40.

Petersen, A.R. (1996) 'Risk and the regulated self: the discourse of health promotion as politics of uncertainty', *Australian & New Zealand Journal of Sociology*, 32, 1: 44–57.

Petersen, A.R. and Lupton, D. (1996) *The New Public Health: Health and self in the age of risk*, London: Sage.

Prior, L. (1995) 'Chance and modernity: accidents as a public health problem', in R. Bunton, S. Nettleton and R. Burrows (eds) *The Sociology of Health Promotion*, New York: Routledge.

Reaves, J.L. and Campbell, R. (1994) *Cracked Coverage: Television News, the Anti-Cocaine Crusade, and the Reagan Legacy*, London: Duke University Press.

Rose, N. (1989) *Governing the Soul: The Shaping of the Private Self*, London: Routledge.

Rose, N. (1993) 'Government, authority and expertise in advanced liberalism', *Economy and Society*, 22, 3: 283–98.

Savage, M., Barlow, J., Dickens, P. and Fielding, T. (1992) *Property, Bureaucracy and Culture: Middle Class Formation in Contemporary Britain*, London: Routledge.

Schrift, A.D. (1995) 'Reconfiguring the subject as a process of self: following Foucault's Nietzschean trajectory to Butler, Laclau/Mouffe, and beyond', *New Formations*, 25: 28–39.

Starr, P. (1982) *The Social Transformation of American Medicine*, New York: Basic Books.

Stevenson, H.M. and Burke, M. (1991) 'Bureaucratic logic in new social movement clothing: the limits of health promotion research', *Health Promotion International*, 6: 281–96.

TIHR (Tavistock Institute of Human Relations) (1956) 'Some psychological and sociological aspects of toilet tissues – final report', document No. 419 (July), London: Tavistock Institute of Human Relations.

Turner, B.S. (1992) 'The interdisciplinary curriculum: from social medicine to postmodernism', in B.S. Turner *Regulating Bodies: Essays in Medical Sociology*, London: Routledge.

Turner, B.S. (1995) *Medical Power and Social Knowledge*, 2nd edition, London: Sage.

Valverde, M. (1996) 'Governing out of habit: from "habitual inebriates" to "addictive personalities"', paper presented to the History of the Present Group, London School of Economics, 22 May.

WHO (World Health Organisation) (1986) *Ottawa Charter for Health Promotion*, Canada: WHO. (Reproduced in *Health Promotion*, 1: 1.)

WHO (World Health Organisation) (1991) *Introducing the Lifestyles and Health Department*, Copenhagen: Regional Office for Europe.

Williams, G. and Popay, J. (1994) 'Lay knowledge and the privilege of experience', in J. Gabe, D. Kelleher and G. Williams (eds) *Challenging Medicine*, London: Routledge.

Index

Page numbers in **bold** denote major section devoted to subject

infertility treatment 6
insanity *see* madness
intelligence tests 68, 69, 83
intersectoral collaboration 195, 197
intertextuality 32–5, 44, 48

Jones, K. 17
journals, medical: risk articles 215

Kant, I.: *The Conflict of the Faculties* 182
Kindergarten Training College (KTC) 85
kindergartens 82–3, **83–6**, 87–9
Klein, Renate 136
knowledge: expert and 'lay' 231–2; and female body 140–1; magazines and medical 232–4, 235, 242; *see also* power/knowledge
KTC (Kindergarten Training College) 85

La Berge, A. 178
Laing, R.D. x, 162
Lalonde, M. 227
language: Foucault on role of 155, 166, 167; and neo-liberalism 185; and personality disorder 57; and self-starvation 163
Lash, S. 190
law: and psychiatry **53–7**, 70
lead 201
liberalism: and health policy 181, 182–5; Rose on features of 225; *see also* advanced liberalism; neo-liberalism
Lunacy Act (1878) 58, 66, 68
lunatics: distinction between idiots and 57–8, 64, 65; treatment of in Australia 58–9; *see also* madness
Lupton, D. xiii, 27, 204
Lupton, D. and Chapman, S. 219
Lush, Mary 83–4, 85
Lyotard, 3, 33–4, 235

McDonaldisation xviii
Macey, David xi
Machiavelli 176, 177
McNay, Lois 43, 152, 154, 165, 167

Macquarie, Governor 58
madness x, 60–1; construction of categories 60–1; and criminality 54–5, 58–60; lower profile of 18, 19; treatment of lunatics in Australia 58–9
Madness and Civilisation ix, x, **16–19**, 20, 26, 53, 101
magazines 242–3; growth in health products 235–6; heterogeneity of 240; and medicine **232–5**; and popular health **231–2**, 242; and self-care 238–9, 241; *see also Good Housekeeping*
market: introduction into healthcare 226–7, 230
Marx, Karl 2, 25, 48
Marxism xi, xii, 95
May, C. 27, 102
medical gaze *see* 'clinical gaze'
medical journals 215
'medical police' 177, 178
medicalisation **144–5**; and objectification of bodies **155–60**
medicalisation critique 5, **94–108**; advocates of 95–7; criticism of 97–8; critiques of Foucauldian perspective 101–6; and doctor–patient relationship 96–7, 98; dominance of 97; emergence 95; and feminists 97, 144, 145; Foucauldian perspective 94, 98–101, 107; solutions 97, 106, 107
medicine 5, 22, 100; and power 95, 96, 97
menopause: and fitness 142; and HRT 135; medicalisation of xii, 139–40, 141
mental defectives 66, 68–9
Mental Defectives Act (1939) 68, 69
mental health x, xiv, xix; categories 55, 60–4; child *see* child mental health; concept of personality *see* personality; law and psychiatry 53–7, 70; new focus on 18; as socially constructed 16–17; *see also* madness; *Madness and Civilization*